The Ultimate Guide to Enhancing Strength, Balance, and Flexibility:70 Chair Exercises for Seniors over 60

The Best Chair Workout for Older Adults To Build Strength, Balance, Flexibility, Joint Health, Improved Mobility, Pain Relief, and Injury Prevention

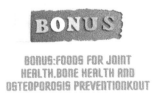

BONUS:FOODS FOR JOINT HEALTH,BONE HEALTH AND OSTEOPOROSIS PREVENTIONKOUT

Adam T Walls

Bonus:Foods for Joint Health,Bone Health and Osteoporosis Prevention:

Essential Nutrients for Strong Bones and Joints

Include Fatty Acids with Omega-3:

An important factor in lowering inflammation and enhancing joint health is omega-3 fatty acids. Omega-3s may be found in abundance in fatty fish such as salmon, mackerel, and sardines, as well as in plant-based foods like walnuts, chia seeds, and flaxseeds. By including these items in your diet, seniors over 60 can improve their mobility and flexibility by reducing joint pain and stiffness.

Eat a Lot of fruits and veggies:

Rich in phytonutrients and antioxidants that reduce inflammation and promote general joint and bone health are colorful fruits and vegetables. Berries, tomatoes, bell peppers, and leafy greens are especially healthy since they are rich in antioxidants, vitamins, and minerals. To receive as much of these vital nutrients as possible from your meals, try to fill half of your plate with fruits and vegetables.

Incorporate Foods High in Calcium:

Particularly as we age, calcium is crucial for keeping healthy bones and avoiding osteoporosis. Although calcium is commonly found in dairy products like milk, yogurt, and cheese, it may also be found in non-dairy foods like tofu, fortified plant-based milks, and leafy greens like collard and kale. Bone health is supported and calcium absorption is improved when vitamin D sources like fatty fish or sunshine exposure are combined with meals high in calcium.

Keep Inflammatory Foods to a Minimum:

Certain foods have the potential to increase bodily inflammation, which can cause joint pain and discomfort. Common causes of inflammation include processed meals, trans fats, refined carbs, and sugary snacks. Seniors over 60 can help reduce inflammation and improve joint health by reducing their intake of these inflammatory foods and opting instead for full, nutrient-dense choices.

Accept Good Fats:

Nuts, seeds, avocados, and olive oil are good sources of healthy fats that help lubricate joints and reduce inflammation. Additionally beneficial to general health and cardiovascular health are these fats. A diet rich in healthy fats can support the preservation of joint flexibility and mobility while supplying vital nutrients for general well-being.

Add some Turmeric to Spice It Up:

Curcumin, a potent substance with anti-inflammatory qualities, is found in turmeric. Turmeric tea or meals prepared with turmeric extract can help reduce stiffness and discomfort in the joints brought on by arthritis and other inflammatory diseases. Turmeric is a beneficial addition to the diet for seniors over 60 since it also promotes bone health and may help avoid osteoporosis.

Select Sources of Lean Protein:

Maintaining muscle mass and promoting general strength and mobility require protein. Pick lean protein foods to provide your body with the building blocks it needs for muscle growth and repair, such as fish, chicken, beans, and lentils. For seniors over 60, including lean protein in meals and snacks can help promote joint health and improve physical activity.

Drink Plenty of Water:

Drinking enough water is crucial for maintaining healthy joints and general wellness.

Water facilitates the lubrication of joints, minimizing friction and providing cushioning during motion. Moreover, it facilitates the delivery of nutrients to tissues and cells, promoting the healing and restoration of muscles. To maintain adequate hydration levels and promote joint health, seniors over 60 should strive to drink at least 8–10 glasses of water each day, and more if they are physically active or live in a hot region.

Table of content

Introduction

This is "The Ultimate Guide to Enhancing Strength, Balance, and Flexibility: 70 Chair Exercises for Seniors Over 60"

Greetings, reader, and welcome to a voyage of vitality and well-being designed only for seniors sixty and older. We will examine the transforming potential of chair exercises in this in-depth tutorial, which is intended to improve flexibility, balance, and strength. This book is your go-to resource for attaining ideal health and vitality, regardless of where you are in your fitness journey or how you want to continue living an active lifestyle.

Strength, balance, and flexibility are crucial for seniors

The preservation of strength, balance, and flexibility becomes more and more important as we age for our general health and well-being. These three elements are essential for maintaining one's independence, avoiding accidents, and improving one's quality of life. Let's examine each of these factors' importance for seniors in more detail:

Strength: Retaining muscular strength is necessary to carry out daily activities on your own, like getting up from a chair, carrying groceries, and climbing stairs. In addition to preserving muscle mass, strength training exercises increase bone density and lower the risk of osteoporosis and fractures. Strong muscles also help seniors maintain an active and involved lifestyle by improving posture, joint stability, and general mobility.

Balance is the cornerstone of mobility and stability. It enables people to walk around securely and keep an erect posture. Decreases in balance with age can raise the chance of falls in seniors, which can lead to major injuries such as fractures, brain traumas, and confidence loss. Exercises for balance will help you keep your balance, strengthen the muscles that support it, enhance your coordination, and lessen your risk of falling. These benefits will help you become more independent and preserve your quality of life.

The range of motion in your joints and muscles is referred to as flexibility, and it's necessary to have this range of motion to carry out daily tasks comfortably and easily. Our muscles and connective tissues tend to stiffen as we age, which reduces our flexibility and raises our risk of injury. Frequent stretching exercises can help prevent these age-related changes by increasing general functional ability, lowering muscular tension, and improving joint mobility. Exercises for flexibility are also very important in preventing musculoskeletal injuries and in treating common conditions like stiffness and back discomfort.

Using Chair Exercises to Their Full Potential for Seniors

In this section, we'll examine the amazing advantages that chair exercises provide seniors, giving them a practical and approachable means of enhancing their strength, flexibility, and balance. Let's take a quick look at the benefits that chair workouts might provide for senior citizens:

Convenience and Accessibility: One of the biggest benefits of chair exercises is that they can be performed by people of various fitness levels and abilities. Chair exercises are a safe, comfortable, and portable solution that can be used anywhere, at home, in a community center, or even on the go. They can be used for injury recovery, chronic disease management, or just for staying active. Chair exercises remove participation barriers by not requiring specific equipment or gym memberships, making training more accessible to elders.

Low-Impact and Joint-Friendly: Seniors with osteoporosis, arthritis, or other musculoskeletal conditions should pay special attention to chair exercises since they are naturally low-impact, putting less strain on the joints and lowering the risk of damage. Chair exercises facilitate the development of strength, balance, and flexibility in individuals while avoiding excessive pressure on joints that are already vulnerable due to their mild movements and controlled resistance. For older persons looking for safe and efficient ways to preserve their physical health and mobility, chair exercises are a great option.

Strength and functional abilities can be significantly increased by regularly engaging in chair exercises, especially for the upper and lower body. Through a range of sitting movements and resistance exercises aimed at specific muscle areas, seniors can improve their functional abilities and carry out daily tasks with more confidence and ease. A stronger body helps seniors preserve their independence and quality of life, which lowers dependency on assistance and improves general well-being. Examples of these activities include lifting groceries and getting in and out of chairs.

Better Balance and Stability: Chair exercises are also very important for seniors to prevent falls and reduce injuries since they improve balance and stability. Older adults can improve the muscles involved in maintaining balance, lower their risk of falling, and increase their confidence in successfully navigating their environment by engaging in specific exercises that test their proprioception and equilibrium. Seniors who include balance-focused exercises in their routine can experience increased mobility, independence, and mental clarity while they go about their everyday lives.

 Enhanced Range of Motion and Flexibility: Last but not least, chair exercises provide an excellent chance to preserve joint mobility and improve flexibility, both of which are essential for maintaining general functional capability and avoiding age-related stiffness and discomfort. Seniors can enhance their range of motion, reduce muscle tension, and improve circulation by adding mild stretching exercises to their routine. This will make them more comfortable and mobile in daily life. Increased flexibility allows seniors to continue being active and involved in the things they love, whether it's reaching up high on a shelf or bending down to tie shoelaces.

In conclusion, chair exercises provide a flexible and powerful means for older adults to become more physically fit, live better, and age with grace and confidence. Older folks can experience increased independence, vigor, and well-being by embracing the advantages of chair workouts, guaranteeing a happy and active existence for years to come.

With the knowledge, resources, and activities included in this extensive guide, seniors will be able to maximize their physical health and overall well-being. This section will provide you with an overview of the book's structure and provide you with tips on how to use it to your fullest advantage.

Comprehending the Organization:

The book starts with an introduction that lays down the foundation for your quest for increased flexibility, balance, and strength. Here's a summary of these elements' significance for seniors and an explanation of how chair exercises can support these objectives.

Body Chapters: The book's main body is broken up into several chapters, each of which focuses on a different facet of health and fitness. These chapters contain thorough explanations of a variety of activities, as well as advice, methods, and adjustments to fit the needs and skills of the individual.

Finally, the book offers a brief overview of the most important lessons learned as well as a last message of support to encourage readers to keep up their commitment to an active and healthy lifestyle.

How to Make Effective Use of It:

Let's begin with the introduction:
Start your adventure by attentively reading the introduction to get a clear idea of the goal and format of the book. Notice the advantages of chair exercises and the good effects they might have on your life.

Determine Your Needs: Spend some time determining your present fitness level, as well as any particular objectives or constraints you may have, before beginning the workouts. This will enable you to modify the routines to suit your own requirements and tastes.

Examine the Body Chapters: Afterwards, concentrate on topics of particular interest or concern as you go through the book's body chapters. Because each chapter is divided into smaller sections, it's simple to navigate and locate the information you require.

Participate in the activities: Read through the activities and take note of the suggested methods and directions. Practice at your own pace and take your time getting acquainted with each exercise.

Tailor Your Program: After you feel confident performing the exercises, think about coming up with a unique program that works for your schedule and fitness objectives. Combine exercises from many chapters to focus on particular body parts and spice up your training.

Finally, keep track of your development over time to see how your strength, balance, and flexibility have improved. For keeping track of your workouts, measurements, and any changes you observe in your general well-being, utilize the accompanying tracking sheets or keep a notebook.

You can make full use of chair exercises to improve your physical health, confidence, and quality of life by adhering to these instructions and actively participating in the book's content. Now, take a seat, settle in, and let's start this journey toward more vigor and health!

Chapter 1:

Understanding the Basics

Knowing the Fundamentals of Senior Chair Exercises

The basic ideas behind chair exercises for seniors will be covered in this section, giving you a strong basis on which to build when implementing these exercises into your daily routine. Gaining a basic grasp of the exercises will help you perform them safely and effectively, maximizing their advantages for your physical health and overall well-being.

The Value of Adequate Warm-Up and Cool-Down Procedures

Chair exercises, like any other type of exercise, need to be properly prepared for and recovered from in order to maximize results and reduce injury risk. It's crucial to warm up properly before working out in order to loosen up your muscles, raise your heart rate gradually, and get your body ready for action. This can involve dynamic motions to engage important muscle groups, range-of-motion exercises, and mild stretches. In a similar vein, spend some time relaxing with deep breathing techniques and light stretching after your workout to assist ease pain in your muscles and increase your range of motion.

The Significance of Correct Form and Method:

When practicing chair exercises, it is important to maintain good form and technique in order to maximize effectiveness and reduce the risk of injury. Throughout each action, pay special attention to your breathing, alignment, and posture. Adjust as necessary to keep your stability and control. Rather than depending just on force or momentum, concentrate on using the right muscles and moving with intention and control. Do not hesitate to ask a certified physical therapist or fitness instructor for advice if you are unclear about the proper technique for a given exercise.

Advice on Choosing a Robust Chair for Workouts:

Your comfort and safety when performing chair exercises can be greatly impacted by the kind of chair you use. To offer a secure foundation for your motions, pick a chair that is strong, steady, and has a straight back and firm support. Steer clear of chairs with arms or wheels that could impair your stability or range of motion. Make sure the chair is the appropriate height for you as well, so that when you sit, your knees should be bent 90 degrees and your feet should rest comfortably on the floor. If required, raise or lower the seat using a cushion or folded towel to get the best possible alignment and comfort.

Knowing these fundamentals of chair workouts for seniors will make it easier and more confident for you to start your fitness journey. Always pay attention to your body's signals, begin cautiously, and as your strength, balance, and flexibility improve, progressively up the intensity and duration of your workouts. Chair exercises can help you maintain your independence, vitality, and activity far into old age if you practice them regularly and with determination.

Evaluating Your Present State of Fitness

It's critical to evaluate your existing fitness level before starting any program in order to establish your starting point, pinpoint areas for growth, and create reasonable goals. We'll look at several easy fitness tests in this area that can help you determine your level of flexibility, balance, and strength. We'll also go over how crucial it is to create realistic goals, recognize your limitations, and monitor your development over time in order to guarantee a secure and fruitful fitness journey.

Easy Strength, Balance, and Flexibility Exercises
Power
Chair Stand Examination:
- Place your feet flat on the ground and take a seat in a firm chair.
- Try to find as many opportunities to stand and sit again in a 30-second period.
- Keep track of how many times you can rise up and then sit back down.
- A higher figure denotes stronger lower body muscles.

Test of Arm Curls:

- Take a seat in a chair and hold a weight (such as cans or water bottles) in each hand.
- Curl the weights toward your shoulders while bending your elbows.
- In 30 seconds, perform as many curls as you can.
- Determine how many curls were accomplished with good form.
- A higher figure denotes stronger upper body muscles.

Equilibrium:
Test of a Single Leg Stand:
- Place your feet hip-width apart while standing behind a chair.
Elevate one foot off the ground while maintaining balance with the other.
- Aim for 30 seconds and hold the position as long as you can.
- Continue with the opposite leg.
- Greater stability and balance are indicated by longer hold periods.

Test of Tandem Walk:
- Step one foot straight ahead of the other, toe to heel.
- Take ten steps forward in a straight line while keeping your balance.
- Retrace your steps and return to the beginning.
- A straight, steady walk suggests that you have superb balance control.

Adaptability
Test of Sitting and Reaching:

- Extend your legs in front of you while sitting on the floor.
Stretch as far forward as you can toward your toes while maintaining a straight knee.
- Measure the distance reached after holding the stretch for a short while.
- Take the best result after repeating the exam twice.
- More distance signifies improved flexibility in the lower back and hamstrings.

Recognizing Your Limitations and Establishing Reasonable Objectives
Recognize Your Body:
- Be truthful with yourself on any physical restrictions or health issues you may be experiencing.
- Before beginning any new fitness regimen, speak with your doctor, particularly if you have any prior injuries or medical issues.

Establish SMART objectives:
Ensure that your objectives are Time-bound, Relevant, Specific, Measurable, and Achievable.
- Concentrate on setting manageable goals that suit your preferences and skill level.
- To monitor progress and maintain motivation, divide more ambitious objectives into smaller, more doable benchmarks.

Monitoring Development Over Time
Maintain a Fitness Diary:

- Keep track of your initial fitness test results and measurements so you can monitor your progress over time.
- Keep a record of your workouts, noting the length, level of difficulty, and any adjustments you make.

As you continue on your fitness adventure, take note of any changes in your strength, balance, flexibility, and general well-being.

Frequent Reevaluation:
- Reevaluate your level of fitness on a regular basis using the same tests and measures.
- To assess your development and pinpoint areas in need of more work, compare your present performance to your baseline.
- Modify your workout plans and goals in response to your changing capabilities and ambitions.

Precautions and Advice for Keeping Secure During Exercise
Pay Attention to Your Body:
- During activity, be mindful of any pain, discomfort, or strange sensations.
- If you feel lightheaded, breathless, have chest pain, or any other worrisome symptoms, stop right once.

Adapt workouts as necessary to your degree of comfort and physical capabilities.

Warm-Up and Dissipate:

- Always warm up gently before beginning an exercise routine to get your body ready for action and lower the chance of damage.
- Use stretches and dynamic motions to improve joint mobility, flexibility, and blood flow.
- To reduce your heart rate, release tight muscles, and encourage relaxation, slowly cool down after your workout.

Employ the Right Tools:
- Wear loose-fitting, comfortable clothes and supportive shoes to promote maximum range of motion.
Make sure there are no risks or obstructions in your workout environment to avoid tripping, falls, or mishaps.
- Make any necessary adjustments or use of assistive technology to ensure stability and safety when exercising.

Remain Fueled and Hydrated:
To keep hydrated and perform at your best before and after exercise, drink lots of water.
Consume a nutrient-rich, well-balanced diet to enhance muscle growth and recuperation after workouts.
To avoid pain and digestion problems, avoid working out right after a large meal or when you're empty handed.

Consult a Professional:
-Take into consideration creating a customized workout program that fits your requirements and goals by

consulting with a licensed fitness instructor, physical therapist, or other healthcare professional.

-To guarantee a secure and productive workout, adhere to their advice regarding the frequency, intensity, and evolution of your exercises.

You can start your fitness journey with confidence by adhering to these recommendations, adding easy fitness tests, establishing reasonable goals, and emphasizing safety precautions. This will ensure that you're taking proactive measures to enhance your strength, balance, flexibility, and general health and well-being. Recall that improvement requires persistence and time, so practice self-compassion and acknowledge your accomplishments as you go.

How to spot injury or overexertion indicators.

Identifying Symptoms of Injury or Overexertion

It's critical to pay attention to your body's signals and know when to slow down, rest, or seek medical assistance when pursuing health and fitness. Pushing too hard, ignoring warning signs, or executing exercises incorrectly can all lead to overexertion and injury. In this section, we'll go over typical indicators of injury and overexertion as well as practical preventative and management techniques.

Symptoms of Excessive Work

Physical Indications:
- Fatigue: Consistently feeling worn out or fatigued, even after getting enough sleep.
- Muscle Weakness: A discernible loss of strength or endurance when working out.
- Increased Heart Rate: Prolonged palpitations or a fast heartbeat following physical activity.
- Shortness of Breath: Having trouble breathing or catching your breath, particularly when exercising.
- Lightheadedness or Dizziness: Experiencing lightheadedness or faintness, especially while standing up or shifting positions.
- Excessive Sweating: Feeling cold or clammy, or sweating a lot.

Signs of Emotion:
- Irritability:bEasily becoming angry, upset, or cranky.
- Decreased Motivation: A decrease in interest or zeal for regular activities or exercise.
- Trouble Concentrating: Incapacity to concentrate or focus on assignments.
- Stress or Anxiety: High levels of stress, anxiety, or worry.

Indications of Damage

Acute Damage:
Sharp Pain: Acute, sharp pain in a particular bodily part that frequently denotes a tear, sprain, or strain.
- Swelling: Outward signs of redness, swelling, or inflammation near a muscle or joint.
- Bruising:nSkin discolouration or bruises that suggest internal bleeding or tissue damage.
- Limited Range of Motion: Pain or stiffness preventing a joint from moving through its whole range of motion.
Instability: The sensation of weakness or instability in a joint, which makes it unsafe to move or bear weight.

Long-Term Damage:
- Persistent Pain: Pain that doesn't go away with rest or medication but instead returns on its own over time.
- Tenderness: Persistent inflammation or irritation indicated by sensitivity to touch in a particular location.
- Stiffness: Extended muscular or joint stiffness or tightness that reduces range of motion and flexibility.
- Reduced Performance: A reduction in functional abilities or athletic performance brought on by persistent pain or discomfort.
- Changes in Movement Patterns:* Modifications to one's gait or compensatory actions taken to ward off discomfort or pain.

Techniques for Management and Prevention

Pay Attention to Your Body:

- During exercise, be aware of your body's mental and physical cues and modify your degree of activity or intensity accordingly.
- Honor the boundaries set by your body and refrain from exerting yourself past the point of exhaustion or discomfort.

Employ the Right Form and Technique:
To lower the chance of injury, concentrate on keeping the right alignment, posture, and technique when performing exercises.
- As your strength and skill level improves, start with lighter weights or resistance and progressively raise the intensity.

Warm-Up and Dissipate:
- Always warm up your muscles and joints thoroughly before starting an exercise routine to get them ready for action.
- After your workout, take a few minutes to cool down to ease muscular pain and aid in healing.

Rest and Convalescence:
- Include rest days in your workout regimen to give your body a chance to heal and regenerate tissues.
- Pay attention to your body's signals when it needs to rest; if necessary, don't be afraid to adjust your workout or take a break.

Consult a Professional:

See a licensed physical therapist, fitness teacher, or other healthcare professional if you have ongoing pain or discomfort when exercising.

- Consult a specialist to create a customized fitness program that takes into account your unique requirements, objectives, and constraints.

Keep Yourself Hydrated and Fed:
- To stay hydrated and sustain peak performance, drink lots of water prior to, during, and following physical activity.

Consume a nutritious, well-balanced diet to aid in the healing and rebuilding of your muscles.

Employ the Right Tools:
To offer support and safety, dress and shoe appropriately for the activity you have selected.

Make sure that any gear or equipment you use is suited to your body correctly and is kept in good condition.

You may maintain a safe and pleasurable exercise routine that promotes your general health and well-being by being proactive in identifying indicators of overexertion or injury and taking appropriate action to prevent and manage these difficulties. To guarantee a great and long-lasting fitness experience, always remember to emphasize self-care, pay attention to your body, and seek professional help when necessary.

The significance of speaking with a healthcare professional before beginning a new fitness program.

It's a commendable move to begin a new workout program, as it can greatly improve your physical and emotional health. To make sure you're starting on a safe and acceptable road towards better health, it's important to speak with a healthcare professional before beginning any new exercise regimen. It is imperative to obtain professional counsel prior to beginning a new workout regimen for the following reasons:

Evaluating Personal Health Status:
Your present state of health, including any injuries, illnesses, or physical restrictions that can affect your capacity to exercise safely, can be evaluated by a healthcare professional. In addition to doing a physical examination and going over any worries or risk factors that might need to be taken care of before beginning an exercise program, they can check your medical history.

Finding Possibile Hazards and Inconsistencies:
Your body's reaction to exercise may be impacted by certain medical conditions or drugs, which could raise the risk of complications or injuries. Before starting a new exercise regimen, a healthcare professional can assist in identifying any potential hazards or inconsistencies that may need to be resolved. Precautions for those with diabetes, heart disease, arthritis, or other long-term medical disorders may be part of this.

Tailoring Exercise Suggestions:

Every person has different exercise objectives, tastes, and health requirements. A medical professional can offer customized workout advice based on your unique requirements and capabilities. They may assist you in selecting suitable activities, establishing reasonable goals, and creating a safe and efficient workout regimen that fits your goals and way of life.

Tracking Development and Making Required Adjustments:
Scheduling routine check-ins with a healthcare provider enables continuous progress tracking and necessary modifications to your workout program. They are able to monitor how your health is changing, assess how you are responding to exercise, and offer suggestions for adjustments or advancement in light of your changing requirements and objectives.

Keeping Accidents and Complications at Bay:
Without the right direction or oversight, beginning a new fitness program can lead to exercise-related injuries and difficulties. By offering advice on suitable warm-up and cool-down routines, suggesting appropriate exercise intensity and duration, and imparting right exercise skills to reduce the chance of injury, a healthcare provider can help prevent injuries.

Offering Encouragement and Assistance:
Support from a healthcare professional can inspire and motivate you to continue your fitness regimen, particularly when things are tough. Along the process,

they can provide direction, responsibility, and comfort, which will help you stay dedicated to your fitness and health objectives.

In conclusion, it is critical to speak with a healthcare professional before beginning any new exercise program in order to maximize your safety, optimize the benefits of your exercises, and foster long-term success in reaching your fitness and health objectives. You can start on a safe and long-lasting fitness path that improves your general well-being and quality of life by collaborating with a healthcare provider.

Chapter 2:

Strength-Building Exercises

Senior Strength-Building Exercises

Any fitness regimen must include strength-building activities, especially for seniors who want to preserve their freedom, mobility, and general quality of life. Strength training can help you reduce the risk of falls, fractures, and other age-related health issues by increasing muscle mass, bone density, joint stability, and functional skills. This section will discuss the value of strength-training activities for seniors and give you a list of some good ones to add to your regimen.

Seniors' Need for Strength-Building Exercises

Maintaining Muscle Mass: Sarcopenia is the term for the normal loss of muscle mass and strength that occurs as we age. By maintaining lean muscle mass, promoting muscle development and maintenance, and halting muscle atrophy, strength-building workouts can halt this decrease.

Enhancing Bone Health: Exercises including strength training also improve bone health by lowering the risk of osteoporosis and fractures and increasing bone density. Seniors may promote bone development and improve their skeletal system by putting their bones through regulated stress with resistance training.

Improving Functional Abilities: Being able to carry out daily duties with confidence and easily depends on having strong muscles and joints. Strengthening exercises help seniors maintain their independence and participation in everyday life by improving functional abilities including walking, climbing stairs, lifting items, and getting in and out of chairs.

Increasing Metabolism and Aiding in Weight Management: Seniors who engage in strength training can maintain a healthy body composition and weight by increasing their metabolic rate and calorie expenditure. Seniors can lower their risk of obesity and associated health issues by increasing their lean muscle mass and improving their energy balance and metabolic efficiency.

Seniors: The Best Strength-Building Exercises

Exercises Using Your Own Bodyweight: - Squats: Place your feet hip-width apart, then raise yourself to a sitting posture by lowering yourself into a chair and back up again.

Lunges: Take a single step forward, lowering your body until your knees are bent 90 degrees. Then, step back to the beginning and repeat on the opposite side.

Push-ups: Work your triceps, shoulders, and chest by performing push-ups on the floor, against a wall, or on a countertop.

Resistance Band Exercises: - Bicep Curls: With your palms facing up, hold a resistance band in each hand. Curl the band towards your shoulders, then carefully drop it back down.

- Tricep Extensions: Raise your arm overhead, stretch your elbow, and then bring yourself back down while holding one end of the resistance band in one hand.

Squat Presses: To activate your quadriceps and hamstrings, place one end of the resistance band under your foot while sitting on a chair. Press your foot forward against the band.

Exercises Using Dumbbells: - Shoulder Press: Raise the weights overhead until the arms are completely extended, then drop them back down. Hold a dumbbell in each hand, palms facing front.

- Chest Press: While lying on your back, grasp a dumbbell in each hand and bend your elbows 90 degrees. Press the weights upward and then downward.

- Deadlifts: Hinge at the hips and lower weights toward the floor while maintaining a straight back, then stand back up with your feet hip-width apart.

Advice for Secure and Successful Strength Training

Start Lightly and Raise Intensity Gradually: As you gain strength and confidence, start with lesser weights or resistance and progressively raise the intensity. Maintaining good form and technique will help you stay injury-free and perform at your best.

Pay Attention to Your Body:
During exercising, pay attention to any pain, discomfort, or strange feelings. If you feel lightheaded, breathless, or have a sharp discomfort, stop right away and seek medical advice if necessary.

Include relax Days: To enable muscles to heal and strengthen, give yourself enough time to recuperate and relax in between strength training sessions. Aim for a minimum of 48 hours of relaxation in between exercises that focus on the same muscle groups.

Remain Hydrated and Nourished: To maintain muscular function and keep hydrated, drink lots of water before, during, and after exercise. Consume a well-balanced meal high in healthy fats, carbs, and protein to support and enhance your exercise and recuperation.

Exercises should be adjusted to your needs and preferences if you have any physical restrictions or ailments. Make use of assistive technology, adjust your range of motion, or select safer and more pleasant workout options.

Seek Professional Advice: To create a customized strength training program that meets your requirements and objectives, think about collaborating with a licensed personal trainer, physical therapist, or other healthcare practitioner. They can offer advice on safe practices, progression, style, and workout choices.

You may benefit from strength training far into your elderly years by adding exercises that increase muscle to your fitness regimen and by paying attention to these safe and efficient training guidelines. Consistency is crucial, so make a commitment to working out regularly and get the benefits of a stronger, healthier, and more resilient body.

Strength of Upper Body

Overview

To execute daily actions like lifting, reaching, and carrying goods, upper body strength is necessary. Increasing the strength of your back, chest, shoulders, and arms can improve your functional skills and general quality of life. We'll look at some efficient upper body strength workouts in this part that you may do at home with basic equipment.

Shoulder rolls and arm circles

Simple yet efficient exercises for warming up the upper body and increasing shoulder mobility and flexibility are arm circles and shoulder rolls. These motions remove tension in the upper back and shoulders, lessen stiffness, and improve blood flow to the muscles.

Arm Circles: - Place your arms at shoulder height straight out to the sides while keeping your feet shoulder-width apart.
- Start by forming little circles with your arms and progressively enlarge them.
- Proceed for ten to fifteen repetitions, then change course and repeat.

Standing with your feet shoulder-width apart and your arms loosely at your sides, perform a shoulder roll.
- Squeeze your shoulders up toward your ears, then back down in a circular motion as you roll them forward.
- After ten to fifteen cycles, switch directions and repeat.

Resistance bands or water bottles for bicep curls
Bicep curls assist in toning and developing the muscles at the front of the upper arm, or biceps. Resistance bands and water bottles are common home objects that may be used for this activity.

Holding water bottles in each hand, palms facing ahead, take a standing position with your feet shoulder-width apart.
Squeeze your biceps by slowly curling the bottles towards your shoulders while keeping your elbows close to your sides.

- Carefully lower the bottles back down, then repeat 10–15 times.

Using resistance bands: - Place the resistance band under your feet, stand with your feet shoulder-width apart, and grip one end in each hand.
- Tension on the band should be maintained as you progressively curl your wrists towards your shoulders while keeping your elbows close to your sides.
- Carefully lower your hands back down, then repeat 10–15 times.

Using the Chair's Edge for Tricep Dips

Tricep dips are a great way to strengthen and define the muscles at the rear of the upper arm, namely the triceps. You may use the edge of a solid chair or bench for this exercise.

Tricep dips: - Take a seat on a chair or bench and place your hands on its edge, fingers pointing front.
- Place your feet in front of you while maintaining a 90-degree bend in your knees and flat feet on the ground.
Bending your elbows to keep them close to your sides, lower your body towards the floor.
- Straighten your arms and contract your triceps to push yourself back up to the starting position.
- Ten to fifteen repetitions should be performed, keeping perfect form the entire time.

You may build total upper body strength and endurance, improve functional abilities, and tone your muscles by using these upper body strength exercises in your workout regimen. As you gain confidence and strength, progressively increase the number of repetitions you begin with.

Strength in the Lower Body

Overview
Strength in the lower body is essential for preserving independence, stability, and mobility as we age. Developing stronger leg, hip, and core muscles can help with balance, coordination, and general functioning ability. We'll look at some great lower body strength exercises in this part that you can do using a chair for support.

Chair Squats Done Correctly
A functional exercise, chair squats work the quadriceps, hamstrings, and glutes in addition to activating the core and stabilizing muscles in the legs. Strength, stability, and mobility in the lower body are enhanced by this exercise.

Chair Squats: - Place yourself in front of a solid chair with your toes pointed forward and your feet hip-width apart to start.
- Lower your body toward the chair as though you were sitting back into it by using your core muscles to hinge at the hips and bending your knees.
- As you descend, maintain an elevated chest, knees in line with your toes, and weight in your heels.
- Lower till your glutes softly touch the chair or until your thighs are parallel to the floor.
- Squeeze your glutes at the peak and push through your heels to get back to the starting position.
- Repeat ten to fifteen times, keeping your form correct the entire time.

Leg Lifts to Develop Your Hamstrings and Quadriceps
Leg lifts serve to increase lower body strength and stability by focusing on the muscles at the front (quadriceps) and rear (hamstrings) of the thigh. You may carry out this workout while seated using a chair for support.

Leg Lifts: - While sitting upright on a chair, place your feet flat on the ground and bend your knees 90 degrees.
- Stretch one leg straight out in front of you and raise it off the ground while maintaining a straight back and a contracted core.
- Hold for a short while before controllingly lowering the leg again.
- Repeat for ten to fifteen repetitions on each side, switching sides, on the other leg.

The calf raises to strengthen the lower legs
The lower leg muscles, or calves, are the focus of calf raises, which enhance balance, strength, and stability. You may do this exercise sitting or standing, supporting yourself if necessary with a chair or wall.

Calf Raises: - Place your feet flat on the floor, hip-width apart, while sitting tall in a chair.
- Raise your body onto your toes by pressing through the balls of your feet to raise your heels off the ground.
- Hold the pose for a few while, then carefully lower your heels back down.
- Concentrate on the tightness in your calf muscles as you repeat for 10 to 15 repetitions.

Using Chair Crunches to Work Your Abdominal Muscles
Targeting the rectus abdominis muscles in the abdomen, seated crunches enhance core stability and strength. You may do this exercise while sitting on a chair and maintaining good posture.

Seated Crunches: – Place your hands behind your head with your elbows sticking out to the sides, and sit tall on a chair with your feet flat on the floor.
- Lift your chest and maintain a straight back by using your core muscles to lean back a little.
- Bring your chest closer to your knees by exhaling as you tighten your abdominal muscles.

Breathe in while keeping your core taut as you make your way back to the beginning position.
- Concentrating on the contraction of your abdominal muscles, repeat for ten to fifteen repetitions.

Twisting Chairs to Exercise Adjacent Muscles
Chair twists assist in increasing core strength, stability, and flexibility by focusing on the obliques, the muscles that run down the sides of the body. You may do this exercise while sitting on a chair and maintaining good posture.

Chair Twists: - Place your hands lightly on your thighs while sitting tall on a chair with your feet flat on the ground.
- Using your core muscles, rotate your body to one side, bringing your knee closer to the opposing shoulder.
Hold for a little period, then go back to the beginning and repeat on the opposite side.
For ten to fifteen repetitions, switch sides while concentrating on your waist's rotation.

Pelvic tilts as a Lower Back Strengthening Exercise
Pelvic tilts serve to enhance posture, strength, and flexibility by focusing on the erector spine, the muscles in the lower back. You may do this workout on the floor or while seated on a chair.

Chapter 3:

Balance Improvement Exercises

Static Equilibrium:

The capacity to keep one's balance when moving in a fixed position is known as static balance. It is an important component of total stability and balance, needed for a variety of tasks from basic everyday living activities to more complicated actions like playing sports and standing straight.

Stretching your spine while seated is a useful technique for enhancing static equilibrium. The erector spinae, one of the muscles that support and maintain the spine, is one of the muscles that are targeted by these stretches. People can improve their posture, which helps with static balance, by strengthening and extending these muscles.

Adding knee raises while seated might also make balance much more difficult. Sitting up, people use their core muscles to balance themselves by elevating one knee at a time. This exercise increases general stability and lowers the risk of falls by strengthening the muscles surrounding the hips and knees in addition to improving balance.

Heel-toe taps are an additional useful exercise for static balance. This is a sitting workout where you alternately tap the toe and heel of one foot. People can enhance their proprioception and coordination, two crucial aspects of static balance, by engaging in this exercise. Regularly performing heel-toe taps can help people gain more control over how their bodies move and posture, which will enhance their stability and balance.

Balance in Motion:

The capacity to keep one's balance while moving or executing dynamic motions is known as dynamic balance. Dynamic balance necessitates the synchronization of several muscle groups to regulate movement and maintain balance in different planes of motion, in contrast to static balance, which concentrates on stability while motionless.

Incorporating rhythmic motions and coordination training can improve dynamic balance. Taking some time to practice your rhythm and coordination might be a fantastic place to start. Simple motions like clapping hands in a rhythmic manner or tapping feet to music can be used for this. Dynamic balance requires proper neuromuscular coordination, which is enhanced by these exercises.

Side leg lifts are an additional useful exercise to improve dynamic balance by testing lateral stability. People who are seated can maintain stability by using their hip and core muscles to elevate one leg to the side. This exercise enhances proprioception and balance control in the lateral plane of motion in addition to strengthening these muscles.

Furthermore, adding leg and arm extensions can improve balance control even further. For this exercise, you must sit and simultaneously stretch one arm and the other leg. People who execute this exercise put their balance and coordination to the test while using a variety of body muscles. Regularly performing arm and leg extensions can help you become more stable overall and have better dynamic balance when performing a variety of functional motions.

In summary, total stability and mobility depend on both dynamic and static balance. People can enhance their stability and posture when standing by combining workouts that focus on static balance, including knee lifts and sitting spine stretches. In a similar vein, adding dynamic balance exercises such as coordination and rhythmic movements helps improve balance stability and control during dynamic movements. Regular use of these exercises can result in notable enhancements to stability, balance, and general functional performance.

equilibrium in function

The capacity to remain steady and under control while engaging in daily tasks and motions is known as functional balance. Functional balance is the capacity to apply balance and stability to tasks in the real world, as opposed to static balance, which concentrates on being steady when stationary, and dynamic balance, which stresses stability while moving.

To carry out daily tasks like walking, ascending stairs, reaching for things, and getting in and out of seats, functional balance is essential. It also has a big impact on leisure activities, work-related duties, and sports performance. In essence, functional balance enables people to move effectively and securely in a variety of settings.

Enhancing functional balance is teaching the body to combine strength, flexibility, balance, and coordination to carry out particular activities efficiently. Exercises and games that replicate the motions and difficulties of everyday living are necessary for this. Exercises that mimic typical motions found in everyday life, such as single-leg stands, squats, lunges, and balancing board activities, can assist improve functional balance.

Proprioceptive training can also be used to enhance functional balance. The body's capacity to perceive its location and motion in space is known as proprioception. People can increase their body awareness and capacity to adapt to shifts in balance demands by including proprioceptive activities, such as standing on uneven surfaces or utilizing wobble boards or stability balls.

Training for functional balance should emphasize agility and coordination as well. Engaging in activities that necessitate multidirectional movements, rapid direction changes, and hand-eye coordination can aid in the development of the abilities required to confidently and steadily navigate various situations and circumstances.

Additionally, tailored functional balancing training should be provided to meet individual requirements and objectives. To lower their risk of falling, older individuals could benefit from workouts that emphasize balance improvement during activities like reaching for things or getting up from a seated posture. Conversely, athletes might need to get training that improves their stability and balance when doing actions unique to their activity.

To sum up, functional balance is critical for preserving autonomy, avoiding accidents, and maximizing performance in a range of settings and activities. People may improve their general quality of life and their functional balance by engaging in a range of workouts and activities that test their strength, flexibility, coordination, proprioception, and balance.

Reaching Exercises: Modeling Actual Motion

Since reaching exercises mimic a typical movement pattern seen in daily life, they are an essential part of functional training. Reaching for items above, over a table, or on the ground is necessary for carrying out a variety of jobs effectively and on your own. People may increase their functional strength, mobility, and flexibility by adding reaching exercises to their workout regimen. This will make daily tasks safer and simpler.

The overhead reach is a useful teaching exercise. This exercise involves standing with your feet shoulder-width apart, stretching both arms aloft, and extending your body toward the ceiling as though you are reaching for a high shelf. After a few seconds of holding the stretch, go back to your starting posture. Enhancing shoulder range of motion, flexibility, and mobility is beneficial for reaching overhead during daily tasks like putting dishes away or reaching for objects on high shelves.

The diagonal reach is an additional useful reaching exercise. With your feet shoulder-width apart and your arms relaxed by your sides, begin in a standing stance. As though you were reaching for something on a counter or table, extend one arm diagonally across your body and towards the other side. After a few seconds of holding the stretch, go back to the beginning and repeat on the opposite side. This exercise helps increase the range of motion and flexibility in the upper body, particularly in the shoulders and upper back, which are frequently used in reaching motions.

Furthermore, adding reaching exercises to a training program helps enhance general coordination and balance. Reaching exercises put people's stability to the test by having them keep their balance while reaching farther, simulating situations in which stability and balance are crucial for averting falls and injuries.

In summary, because reaching exercises replicate normal movement patterns found in daily life, they are a crucial part of functional training. Reaching exercises can help people increase their functional strength, flexibility, and mobility, which will make it safer and simpler for them to carry out daily chores on their own.

Using Support to Get Up from a Seated Position and Increase Functional Mobility

Maintaining freedom and mobility in daily life requires the fundamental movement ability to stand up from a sitting posture with assistance. Coordination, strength, and stability in the lower body and core muscles are needed for this exercise. Individuals can preserve their functional independence and enhance their ability to do this necessary action by practicing getting up from a sitting posture with assistance.

The chair stand exercise is a useful exercise to practice standing from a sitting position with assistance. To begin this exercise, place your feet flat on the floor and bend your knees to a 90-degree angle while seated on a firm chair. For support, place your hands on the chair's seat or armrests. To stand up, elevate your chest and maintain a straight back by using your core muscles and applying pressure through your heels. After standing, take a little break before controllingly lowering yourself back to a sitting posture. Carry out the motion many times.

Strengthening the lower body with support while sitting down will assist in strengthening the quadriceps, hamstrings, and glutes—all of which are necessary for executing this exercise. It also improves stability and balance by making it harder for people to lose control while getting up from a sitting to a standing posture.

Additionally, varying the chair stand exercise by adding weight or doing it on unsteady surfaces like a foam pad or balancing cushion will further test the muscles and enhance functional mobility in general.

To sum up, being able to stand up from a seated position with assistance is a basic motor ability that is necessary to preserve one's freedom and mobility in day-to-day activities. People may increase their lower body strength, stability, and balance by performing this exercise regularly and varying it to test their muscles.

This will enhance their capacity to carry out necessary jobs and activities on their own.

Strolling in Place While Seated: Encouraging Balance and Circulation

To enhance circulation, balance, and general physical activity levels, a simple yet effective exercise that can be done practically any place is walking in place while seated. People who are recovering from surgery or injuries, office workers, people with restricted mobility, or anybody who spends a lot of time sitting down will find this low-impact exercise very helpful.

Sit comfortably in a chair with your feet flat on the ground to execute walking in place while seated. Start by raising one foot just a little bit off the ground. Then, in a controlled manner, raise and lower your legs in succession to simulate walking. After a certain amount of time, keep doing this exercise regimen, progressively lengthening it as your endurance increases.

By using the lower body muscles and enhancing blood flow to the legs and feet, walking in place while seated aids with circulation. This might lessen the chance of developing circulation-related problems like blood clots or edema and assist ease the stiffness and pain brought on by extended sitting.

Additionally, by forcing people to maintain stability during the walking action, sitting-related walking might enhance balance and coordination. The proprioceptive system and core muscles are engaged during this workout, which is crucial for preserving stability and balance throughout regular tasks.

Walking in place while seated has several cardiovascular advantages; however, adding arm motions, such as swinging the arms back and forth in time with the leg movements, can further increase these benefits and give a full-body exercise.

In summary, walking in place while seated is an easy-to-achieve exercise that has several advantages for enhancing circulation, enhancing balance, and raising levels of physical activity. Regardless of age or degree of fitness, people may improve their general health and well-being by adding this activity to their regular regimen.

Exercises that increase flexibility are crucial for preserving general mobility, avoiding injuries, and enhancing functional movement patterns. This chapter concentrates on certain exercises that target major muscle groups to improve the range of motion and reduce tension, with the goal of increasing flexibility in both the upper and lower body.

Flexibility of the Upper Body:

Using Your Neck to Release Tension:

Neck stretches are a great method to reduce stress and increase cervical spine flexibility. A simple neck stretch may be done by sitting or standing tall and relaxing your shoulders. Till a slight strain is felt along the side of the neck, slowly bend the head to one side and bring the ear towards the shoulder. Repeat on the other side after holding the stretch for 15 to 30 seconds. This exercise relieves tension in the neck muscles, which lessens soreness and stiffness.

Stretches for the Shoulders to Increase Range of Motion:

By focusing on the muscles and connective tissues that surround the shoulder joint, shoulder stretches help to improve flexibility and range of motion. The cross-body shoulder stretch is a useful exercise for the shoulders. To begin, spread one arm shoulder-width across the torso. Press the arm gently toward the chest with the other hand until the upper back and shoulder start to expand. Repeat on the opposite side after holding the stretch for 15 to 30 seconds. This stretch relieves shoulder tension, particularly after extended hours of sitting or computer work.

Stretching Your Chest Opener to Avoid Hunching Over:

Stretching the muscles in the chest and front shoulder helps offset the consequences of hunching over and having a bad posture. Place your feet hip-width apart and stand tall to complete this stretch. Raise the arms away from the body, elevate the hands behind the back, and press the shoulder blades softly together. Feel a deep stretch over the chest and front of the shoulders as you hold the pose for 15 to 30 seconds. By opening up the chest and enhancing posture, this exercise eases the strain and pain brought on by stooping.

Flexibility of the Lower Body:

Leg extension and seated hamstring stretch:

The hamstrings, which are frequently tense from extended sitting or physical activity, are the focus of the seated hamstring stretch. Sit on a chair's edge with one leg straight out in front of you and the other foot flat on the ground to complete this stretch. Up until a slight strain is felt along the back of the extended leg, maintain a straight back and bend forward at the hips. After holding the stretch for 15 to 30 seconds, swap your legs. This exercise promotes improved posture and lowers the risk of lower back discomfort by increasing hamstring flexibility.

Stretching the Quadriceps While Seated:

The muscles at the front of the thigh, which might grow tense from activities like walking, jogging, or cycling, are the focus of the quadriceps stretch. Sit upright on a chair with your feet flat on the ground to complete this stretch. After grabbing one ankle, slowly bring the heel toward the glutes until the front of the thigh stretches. After holding the stretch for 15 to 30 seconds, swap your legs. This exercise promotes improved knee function and lowers the chance of injury by increasing quadriceps flexibility.

Stretching Your Calf Using the Chair as Support:

The gastrocnemius and soleus muscles, which can get tense from activities like walking, jogging, or wearing high heels, are among the lower leg muscles that are targeted by the calf stretch. As you stand facing a chair or wall for support, complete this stretch. Reposition one foot such that the knee is straight and the heel remains on the ground. Feel the rear leg's calf stretch as you slant forward a little. After holding the stretch for 15 to 30 seconds, swap your legs. This exercise helps increase calf muscle flexibility, which enhances ankle mobility and lowers the chance of injury.

Exercises that increase flexibility are crucial for preserving general mobility and avoiding injuries, to sum up. Stretching exercises for the upper and lower body can help people increase their range of motion, relieve stress, and improve their posture and movement patterns. People of all ages and fitness levels may practice these exercises since they are easy to learn and can be done practically any place with minimum equipment. They are also simple but effective.

Whole-Body Adaptability:

Exercises for full-body flexibility work several muscle groups at once, increasing functional movement patterns and fostering general mobility. Stretches targeting different body parts can help people become more flexible from head to toe, enabling them to move with grace and ease throughout everyday activities. Three essential full-body flexibility exercises that stretch the entire body and improve flexibility overall are the main topics of this chapter.

Spinal Twist on a Chair:

A great exercise to stretch your entire back and increase spinal mobility is the sitting spinal twist. Sit upright on the floor with your legs straight out in front to complete this stretch. With the foot flat on the floor outside the opposing thigh, bend one knee and cross it over the other leg. Put one hand behind the torso for stability and the other on the bent knee for support. Take a deep breath to stretch the spine, and release it as you slowly rotate your body in the direction of your bent knee, supporting yourself with the arm on the other side. After holding the stretch for 15 to 30 seconds, swap sides. This exercise relieves stiffness in the spine, increases spinal mobility, and releases tension in the back muscles.

Bending Forward While Seated:

Targeting the hamstrings and lower back, the sitting forward bend increases flexibility in these vital regions. Sit upright on the floor with your legs straight out in front to complete this stretch. Breathe in to stretch the spine; exhale as you bend forward at the hips and extend your hands to your toes. As you bend forward, keep your back straight and your chest up, bringing your chest closer to your thighs. Feel a deep stretch throughout the lower back and back of the legs as you hold the pose for 15 to 30 seconds. This exercise promotes improved posture, lessens lower back strain, and increases hamstring flexibility.

Side Stretch While Seated:

The sitting side stretch increases lateral flexibility and mobility by focusing on the muscles along the sides of the body. Sit upright on the floor with your legs straight out in front to complete this stretch. Breathe in to stretch your spine; when you extend one arm above to the other side, release the breath. To provide stability, keep the other hand firmly placed on the floor and refrain from bringing your chest close to your thighs. Feel a deep stretch down the side of the body from the fingers to the hips as you hold the pose for 15 to 30 seconds. This exercise helps release tension in the side body, enhance the range of motion in the spine, and improve lateral flexibility.

To sum up, full-body flexibility exercises are critical for improving functional movement patterns, reducing injury, and boosting general mobility. Through the integration of stretches such as the sitting side stretch, seated forward bend, and seated spinal twist into a consistent exercise regimen, people may enhance their overall flexibility, guaranteeing effortless and graceful movement during their everyday routines. These exercises are accessible to everyone looking to increase their flexibility and general well-being since they are straightforward yet effective, and they can be tailored to accommodate people of different ages and fitness levels.

Chapter 5:

Advanced Chair Exercises: Using Creativity to Improve Fitness
For people who prefer sitting workouts or have restricted mobility, chair exercises provide an adaptable and convenient means to increase fitness and mobility. To improve total strength, flexibility, and cardiovascular fitness, this chapter covers advanced chair exercises that integrate compound motions, yoga flows, aerobics, and Pilates-inspired exercises.

Compound Movements: To complete a single exercise, several joints and muscle groups must cooperate. Compound motions can enhance chair exercises' efficiency and efficacy by enabling users to work many muscle groups at once and enhance their general strength and coordination. The sitting chair yoga flow sequence is one type of compound chair workout.

Sequence for a Seated Chair Yoga Flow:

With the use of a sitting chair yoga flow sequence, people may enhance their flexibility, balance, and sense of calm while seated and reap the health benefits of yoga. Usually, this sequence consists of a series of chair-adapted flowing motions, breathwork, and meditation exercises. Seated forward bends, mild twists, side stretches, and seated cat-cow stretches are common postures in a seated chair yoga flow sequence. These exercises encourage relaxation, lessen stress and tension in the body and mind, and assist in enhancing flexibility in the shoulders, hips, and spine.

Chair Aerobics: Using arm and leg motions, chair aerobics is a dynamic type of exercise that increases heart rate and enhances cardiovascular fitness while seated. Those with restricted mobility or those recuperating from surgery or an accident who might not be able to participate in conventional aerobic exercises can particularly benefit from this kind of exercise. Chair aerobics usually consists of a series of exercises that are meant to enhance circulation and raise heart rate, such as arm circles, sitting jumping jacks, and seated marching. Chair aerobics focuses on the cardiovascular system, muscles, and joints while combining arm and leg motions to offer a full-body workout that enhances general fitness and well-being.

Chair Exercises Inspired by Pilates:

Chair exercises with Pilates influence target alignment, strength, and stability in the core and apply the concepts of Pilates to enhance posture and practical movement patterns. To increase strength, flexibility, and control, these exercises usually focus on the core muscles, which include the back, obliques, and abdominals. sitting pelvic tilts, sitting spine twists, seated leg circles, and seated abdominal curls are examples of common Pilates-inspired chair exercises. Through the use of Pilates concepts like breath control, attention, and accuracy, these exercises assist people in strengthening and stabilizing their core, correcting their posture, and improving their general body awareness and control.

To sum up, advanced chair workouts provide a fun and practical approach to improving your mobility and fitness while seated. People can enhance strength, flexibility, cardiovascular fitness, and general well-being by adding Pilates-inspired exercises, chair yoga flows, chair aerobics, and complex motions into a regular workout regimen. These exercises are a great resource for anybody trying to get healthier and fitter while sitting down since they can be customized to match the requirements and skills of people of different ages and fitness levels.

Resistance Exercise

Resistance Training: Developing Power and Stamina

Resistance training, sometimes referred to as weight training or strength training, is a type of exercise in which resistance is used to test the muscles, increase strength, and develop endurance. This chapter covers a variety of resistance training techniques, such as using household objects as weights, resistance bands, and safe methods for gradually building up resistance.

Resistance Bands Added for an Added Challenge:

Workouts may be made more challenging and varied by using resistance bands, which are handy and portable instruments that can be used in several resistance training routines. Because these bands are available in several resistance levels, users may progressively up the intensity of their workouts as they get better.

Resistance bands have the benefit of offering varying resistance throughout the range of motion, which can enhance strength and muscle activation more successfully than standard weights alone. Resistance bands also provide you with a greater range of motion and may be used in different ways to stimulate different muscle areas.

Exercises with resistance bands include leg lifts, squats, shoulder presses, chest presses, and bicep curls. People may successfully target main muscle groups, increase muscular strength and endurance, and improve overall fitness and performance by adding resistance bands into a regular strength training practice.

Using Common Household Items as Weights, such as Cans or Water Bottles:

Household objects like water bottles, cans, or books can also be utilized as improvised weights for strength training exercises in addition to resistance bands. These products offer a handy and affordable substitute for standard dumbbells or barbells, enabling resistance training for people without access to gym equipment.

Simply grip the object firmly in each hand and do workouts like lunges, overhead presses, bicep curls, and shoulder lifts to use everyday items as weights. You may change the weight by adding or removing water from the containers or by utilizing a combination of objects to progressively increase resistance.

Even though household objects might not offer as much resistance as conventional weights, they can nonetheless efficiently work the muscles and increase strength and stamina—especially for novices or people trying to stay active while not at the gym.

How to Gradually Raise Resistance Safely:

It's crucial to gradually increase resistance when adding resistance training to a fitness regimen to prevent injury and encourage improvement over time. Without overtaxing them, the muscles may adapt and get stronger with a safe increase in resistance.

Gradually increasing workout intensity, length, or frequency is one way to properly increase resistance. As strength increases, this can be achieved by increasing the number of repetitions, sets, or resistance used in the exercises, or by moving on to increasingly difficult versions of the same exercises.

It's also critical to pay attention to your body's signals of exhaustion or pain. To avoid damage, it can be essential to lessen the resistance or alter the action if an exercise seems excessively difficult or painful.

To sum up, resistance training is an important part of a comprehensive fitness regimen that may enhance general health, strength, and endurance. People may safely increase resistance over time, utilize household items as weights, and integrate resistance bands to successfully test their muscles and reach their fitness objectives while reaping the advantages of a stronger, more robust body.

Managing Difficulties

Challenges of Equilibrium: Increasing Stability and Sync

Any comprehensive exercise program should include balance tasks since they enhance proprioception, coordination, and stability. To improve general balance and functional movement patterns, this chapter tackles a variety of balancing difficulties, such as increasing instability using a folded towel or balance cushion, doing eyes-closed activities, and combining single-leg balance exercises with support.

Using a Folded Towel or Balance Cushion to Add Instability:

Using a balancing cushion or folded towel to introduce instability to standard workouts is a useful approach to test balance. Because of the unequal base of support created by these unstable surfaces, the body is compelled to use stabilizing muscles, which enhances balance and coordination.

For instance, to maintain stability and correct form when executing squats or lunges on a folded towel or balancing cushion, the lower body and core muscles must be activated more. Similar to this, challenging stability and enhancing general body control may be achieved by doing upper body workouts like push-ups and shoulder presses with hands resting on a balancing cushion.

People can improve proprioception—the body's sense of its location and movement in space—and balance and coordination in a variety of functional activities by adding instability to their training regimens.

Exercises to Test Proprioception with Closed Eyes:

Using your eyes closed during balancing exercises is another useful strategy to test your proprioception and enhance your coordination and balance. When the eyes are closed, the body is deprived of visual information and is compelled to rely more on proprioceptive feedback from the joints, muscles, and inner ear to stay balanced.

The single-leg balance stance is one easy eyes-closed exercise. Shut your eyes and stand on one leg while concentrating on being steady and in control for a certain amount of time, like thirty to sixty seconds. Since the body adapts to positional changes without the aid of visual signals, this exercise helps enhance proprioception and balance.

Dynamic exercises that include walking or marching while closing one's eyes can also test proprioception and improve balance and coordination in contexts where visual cues may be few or obstructed.

Exercises for Single-Leg Balance with Support:

Exercises for single-leg balance that require assistance are a good method to increase stability and balance while progressively getting harder. To begin, take a position next to a wall or other solid surface for support. Then, raise one foot off the ground and balance on the other leg while keeping your alignment and posture correct.

As your balance gets better, progressively lessen the support by using your fingers to lightly touch the wall or surface, or by utilizing a chair or railing for minimum support. Eventually, work on single-leg balancing exercises without assistance, emphasizing extended periods of stability and control.

People can increase proprioception, strengthen stabilizing muscles, and improve general balance and stability by gradually testing single-leg balance with support. This lowers the chance of falling and improves performance in a variety of daily tasks.

To sum up, balancing difficulties is vital for enhancing proprioception, stability, and coordination—all of which are important for general health and functional movement patterns. People can improve their everyday performance, lower their risk of injury, and increase their balance and coordination by doing single-leg balancing exercises with support, introducing instability using balance cushions or towels, and engaging in eyes-closed exercises.

Chapter 6

Seniors' Daily Chair Exercise Program

Seniors must continue to be physically active in order to preserve their health and mobility. However, due to mobility limitations or health concerns, regular exercise regimens may be difficult for a large number of older persons. For seniors looking to maintain their fitness levels and keep active, chair workouts provide a secure and efficient option. This is an example of a daily chair exercise program designed with seniors in mind. It also includes advice on how to modify programs to meet the requirements and goals of each individual and stresses the significance of consistency in achieving results.

A Daily Chair Exercise Schedule Example:

1. March while seated: Place your feet flat on the ground and take a comfortable seat on a firm chair. Raise one leg to your chest and then return it to its lower position. Continue on the opposite side. For one to two minutes, keep switching up your legs.

2. Chair Yoga Stretch: Take a tall seat, take a deep breath, and raise your arms above your head. Stretch

across the side of your body and gradually tilt to one side as you release the breath. After a few breaths of holding, move back to the middle and repeat on the opposite side. On each side, repeat 3–5 times.

3. Seated Leg Lifts: Place your feet flat on the floor and sit closer to the front edge of your chair. Using your thigh muscles, extend one leg straight out in front of you and then raise it a few inches off the ground. After a little period of time, release your leg. Continue on the opposite side. 10–15 repetitions of each leg should be the goal.

4. Arm Circles: Assume a tall posture, placing your arms at your sides and your feet flat on the ground. Make slow, little circles with your arms in front of you and then progressively larger ones. After ten to fifteen circles, change course and do backward circles with your arms. For one to two minutes, repeat.

5. Seated Side Leg Raises: Place your feet flat on the floor and sit tall in your chair. If necessary, use the chair's sides as support. Maintaining your leg straight and using your outer thigh muscles, raise one leg out to the side. After a little period of time, release your leg. Continue on the opposite side. 10–15 repetitions on each side should be the goal.

6. Seated Torso Twists: Place your feet flat on the floor and sit up straight in your chair. For support, rest your hands on your thighs or the chair's sides. While

maintaining your head in line with your spine, slowly rotate your torso to one side. Hold for a little while before twisting to the opposite side and returning to the middle. Five to ten repetitions for each side.

7. Seated Shoulder Shrugs: Keep your arms at your sides and your feet flat on the ground as you sit tall. Raise your shoulders to your ears and then let them drop back down. Do this ten to fifteen times.

Adapting Routines to Specific Requirements and Objectives:

Since every senior has different skills, limits, and objectives, it's critical to adapt chair exercise programs to meet those needs. The following advice relates to customization:

Speak with a healthcare provider: Seniors should speak with their healthcare provider before beginning any fitness program to be sure the activities are safe and suitable for their particular requirements and medical problems.

Concentrate on particular areas: Seniors can tailor their chair workout regimens to concentrate on particular body parts, such as muscular tone, flexibility, or balance, that they wish to build or enhance.

Exercise modifications: Seniors can make exercises more accessible by altering them if they are too difficult or painful. They can, for instance, use smaller weights, restrict their range of motion, or carry out standing exercises while seated.

Gradually increase intensity: Seniors can incorporate more difficult exercise variants, use heavier weights, or add more repetitions to their chair exercise regimen as they get more used to it.

The Value of Reliability in Observing Outcomes:

If you want to see benefits from chair workout regimens, consistency is crucial. Seniors who want to maintain their fitness levels and observe increases in their strength, flexibility, and general health should try to undertake their chair exercises often, ideally daily. For the following reasons, maintaining consistency is crucial:

Strengthens and extends muscle: Regular chair exercises assist seniors extend their muscular strength and endurance, which can enhance their capacity to carry out everyday tasks and lower their risk of falls and accidents.

Prevents stiffness and enhances range of motion: Seniors who exercise regularly are able to keep their joints flexible and mobile, which can help them avoid stiffness.

Promotes general health: Seniors who engage in chair exercises might benefit from a number of health advantages, such as enhanced mood, improved cardiovascular health, and a lower chance of developing chronic illnesses like diabetes and heart disease. To enjoy these advantages and continue to have the best possible health and wellness, consistency is necessary.

In conclusion, elders may maintain their fitness levels, stay active, and enhance their general health and well-being by engaging in a regular chair exercise regimen designed just for them. Seniors may reap the numerous advantages of persistent exercise far into old age by personalizing routines to meet their unique requirements and goals and by maintaining a regular exercise schedule.

Weekly Timetable

Creating a Weekly Exercise Program That Is Balanced

A weekly workout routine that is well-rounded is necessary to achieve the best possible fitness and health results. People may maximize their outcomes and reduce the risk of injury by combining diversity and advancement, balancing strength, balance, and flexibility exercises, and allocating enough rest and recovery days. Here's a how-to guide for creating a weekly workout routine that incorporates these ideas.

Diversity and Advancement:

Exercise regimen diversity not only keeps people from becoming bored but also guarantees that various muscle groups are used and overall fitness is raised. Progression is also necessary to keep the body challenged and encourage adaptability. Here's how to make your weekly routine more varied and progressive:

Change up the way you exercise:
Throughout the week, alternate between several exercise regimens, including aerobic, strength, flexibility, and balancing activities. Exercises like yoga, Pilates, walking, swimming, resistance band exercises, and bodyweight workouts may fall under this category.

Increase intensity gradually: To encourage advancement, progressively boost the duration, resistance, or intensity of your exercises over time. This might be raising the weight in your strength training routines, lengthening or intensifying your aerobic workouts, or progressing to increasingly difficult yoga positions.

Modify your regimen: To keep your body guessing and avoid plateaus, change up your regimen every few weeks. Experiment with different workout patterns like circuit training, interval training, or HIIT (high-intensity interval training). You may also try new exercises and change the sequence in which you perform your workouts.

Exercises for Balancing Strength, Balance, and Flexibility:

Strength, balance, and flexibility exercises should all be included in a well-rounded weekly exercise program to increase general fitness and lower the chance of injury. Here's how to keep these components under check during the workweek:

Strength training: Try to incorporate two or three sessions of strength training per week, concentrating on the major muscular groups. Exercises like squats, lunges, push-ups, rows, and overhead presses with body weights, dumbbells, or resistance bands may fall under this category.

Exercises for balance: As we age, stability and coordination become increasingly important for both functional mobility and injury prevention. Include balance exercises in your program to help with these issues. This might involve balance-challenging yoga poses, heel-to-toe walks, single-leg stands, and balance board exercises.

Work on your flexibility: To increase your range of motion and avoid stiffness, don't forget to do flexibility exercises. At least twice or three times a week, one should perform stretching exercises that target all of the major muscle groups. Think about planning time in your calendar for yoga, Pilates, or other stretching exercises.

Days of Rest and Recuperation:

For best effects, rest and recuperation days are equally as crucial as activity days. Allowing your body to rest lowers the chance of overtraining and injury, promotes muscle growth and repair, and lessens the likelihood of burnout. You may arrange rest and recuperation days into your weekly routine by following these steps:

Plan at least one day per week for complete relaxation: Every week, set aside one day to give your body a total break from organized activity so that it may heal. On this day, unwind, do light exercises like stretching or walking, and concentrate on self-care techniques like massage or foam rolling.

Pay attention to your body.
Throughout the week, pay attention to how your body feels and modify your routine as necessary. Take an additional day off work or choose to work out at a lesser level if you're feeling worn out or sore.

Make sleep and nutrition a priority: To promote healing and general health, make sure you get enough sleep and eat a healthy diet in addition to taking rest days. Aim for seven to nine hours of sleep every night and feed your body a well-balanced diet high in whole foods, healthy fats, lean protein, and complex carbs.

In summary, the secret to reaching the best fitness and health results is creating a well-balanced weekly exercise program that involves rest and recovery days, strength, balance, and flexibility exercises, and variation and advancement. You may design an exercise program that is sustainable and supports long-term health and well-being by adhering to these recommendations and paying attention to your body's demands.

Monthly Advancement

Monthly Progress: Monitoring, Modifying, and Honoring Accomplishments

Maintaining momentum toward reaching health and fitness objectives requires tracking results and modifying exercise regimens on a monthly basis. People may keep themselves motivated and sustain momentum in their fitness journey by keeping track of their progress, creating new objectives based on improvements, and celebrating their accomplishments. Here's a plan to help you include monthly progression into your workout regimen.

Monitoring Development and Making Modifications:

1. Keep a Workout notebook: Record your workouts in a workout notebook, including the exercises, sets, repetitions, weights, and any comments or observations

regarding your post-workout and during workout feelings. This will enable you to see trends, monitor your development over time, and decide whether to change your routine.

2. Measurements and Evaluations: Make routine measurements and evaluations of important fitness parameters, including cardiovascular fitness, strength, endurance, flexibility, and body weight. This can involve taking a waist circumference measurement, monitoring changes in body fat percentage, testing one's strength through one-repetition maximums, or evaluating one's flexibility with targeted range-of-motion tests.

3. Make Use of Technology: Track your progress and gather information on your workouts, diet, sleep patterns, and other health-related parameters by using fitness applications, wearable technology, or internet resources. Progress charts, goal-setting, and reminders are just a few of the features that many applications and gadgets provide to keep you motivated and accountable.

4. Listen to Your Body: Observe how your exercises affect your body's sensations and reactions. Your present program may need to be adjusted if you consistently feel tired, sore, or don't see any progress. To maximize outcomes and avoid fatigue or injury, be adaptable and willing to make any adjustments to your strategy.

Creating New Objectives in Light of Improvements:

1. Consider Your Progress: At the conclusion of every month, give yourself some time to consider your advancements and successes. Honor successes, point out opportunities for development, and note any difficulties or roadblocks that may have occurred.

2. Reevaluate Your Objectives: Review your objectives in light of your development and present level of fitness to see if any changes or revisions are required. This might include modifying current goals, creating new short- or long-term objectives, or rearranging priorities in response to evolving circumstances or passions.

3. SMART Goal Setting: To guarantee responsibility and clarity, set SMART objectives, which are specific, measurable, attainable, relevant, and time-bound. Divide more ambitious objectives into more manageable chunks, and set deadlines for reaching each benchmark.

4. Push Yourself: Make objectives that will force you to step outside of your comfort zone and push yourself to keep improving. This might include working out for longer periods of time or at a higher intensity, learning new techniques or activities, or taking part in competitions or events that encourage you to stick to your fitness regimen.

Honoring Success and Maintaining Motivation:

1. Acknowledge Progress: No matter how tiny, take the time to acknowledge your victories and accomplishments. Acknowledge the hard work and commitment you've made to your fitness journey and acknowledge your accomplishments as you go.

2. Reward Yourself: Give yourself non-food incentives that are consistent with your values and interests when you accomplish milestones or attain objectives. This may be getting a massage for yourself, purchasing new exercise equipment, or engaging in a pastime or activity that you enjoy.

3. Find Social Support: Assemble a network of friends, family, or exercise partners who will encourage, support, and hold you responsible for your objectives. You may maintain your motivation and social network by joining an exercise group, going to group courses, or engaging in online groups.

4. Visualize Success: Envision reaching your objectives and picture the sensation of doing so. To stay motivated, concentrated, and psychologically ready to tackle difficulties and roadblocks, employ visualization tactics.

To sum up, incorporating monthly progression into your exercise regimen entails monitoring your progress, modifying your plan in response to gains, creating new objectives, and acknowledging your accomplishments. You may keep up the pace in your fitness journey and move closer to your health and fitness objectives by being responsible, adaptable, and driven.

Chapter 7

Chair Exercises with Mindfulness: Improving Well-Being with Mindful Movement

The role that mindfulness plays in enhancing general well-being has come to light more and more in recent years, especially when it is coupled with physical exercise. Chair exercises and other mindful movements provide a special chance to practice mindfulness while exercising, which has several physical and mental health advantages. In the sections that follow, we will examine how to practice mindfulness while performing chair exercises, emphasizing body awareness and breath, as well as the advantages of integrating exercise and mindfulness for general well-being.

Moving With Awareness:

While exercising, mindful movement entails focusing awareness and attention on the here and now. By encouraging people to concentrate on their body alignment, breathing, and movement sensations, this exercise helps people establish a stronger mental-physical bond. Chair exercises are a great way for people of all ages and fitness levels, including the elderly and those with mobility issues, to practice mindful movement since they offer a flexible and accessible platform.

Being Aware While Doing Chair Exercises:

1. Concentrate on Breath: As you execute chair exercises, start by paying attention to your breath. Take note of your breathing pattern, the feeling of air entering and leaving your body, and the rise and fall of your abdomen or chest. Throughout the workout, use your breath as a grounding force to help you stay focused and in the present.

2. Body Awareness: Throughout each exercise, be mindful of the feelings in your body. Take note of the muscles that are used, the joints' range of motion, and any sore or tense spots. Sustain a soft, impartial consciousness of your body's motions, permitting oneself to move effortlessly and smoothly.

3. Remain Present: Make an effort to focus on the here and now while letting go of outside distractions and daydreaming thoughts. If your thoughts stray, gently return them to the movements and breathing sensations to ground yourself in the here and now.

Advantages of Exercise and Mindfulness Together:

1. Less Stress and Anxiety: By encouraging relaxation, lowering the nervous system, and enhancing sentiments of peace and well-being, mindful movement can aid in the reduction of stress and anxiety. Chair exercises can help people become more attentive to their bodily feelings and improve their stress management skills by emphasizing breath and body awareness.

2. Better Focus and Concentration: By teaching the mind to remain alert and present, mindfulness activities can improve focus and concentration. Beyond the physical workout, this can enhance mental clarity, productivity, and cognitive performance throughout the day.

3. Strengthened Mind-Body Connection: Mindful movement cultivates a stronger mental-physical bond that enhances self-awareness, self-control, and embodied presence. People's general well-being can be enhanced by this greater awareness, which can help them comprehend their bodies' requirements and react to bodily sensations properly.

4. Greater Pleasure from Exercise: Adding mindfulness to chair exercises can increase the pleasure and satisfaction derived from physical activity. Exercise may bring people more happiness and joy if they approach it with an inquisitive, nonjudgmental mindset and concentrate on the experience of the moment.

In summary, the integration of mindfulness with chair exercises presents a significant chance to improve overall well-being via deliberate movement. Chair exercises help people develop more mindfulness, lower their stress and anxiety levels, sharpen their focus and concentration skills, and strengthen their mind-body connection by having them practice breath and body awareness. In the end, integrating mindfulness with exercise can result in a more comprehensive approach to health and wellbeing, fostering vigor in the body, mind, and emotions.

Techniques for Reducing Stress

Stress Reduction Methods: Improving Health with Chair Yoga and Relaxation

Stress has become a typical occurrence for many people in today's fast-paced society, negatively affecting both mental and physical health. On the other hand, including stress-reduction strategies in everyday living can lessen the harmful consequences of stress and enhance general well-being. These methods include deep breathing, chair yoga positions, guided visualization, and relaxation exercises. Here, we look at how incorporating these techniques into everyday activities might help people feel less stressed and more at ease.

Inhaling deeply:

Deep breathing, sometimes referred to as belly breathing or diaphragmatic breathing, is an easy yet effective method for lowering tension and encouraging calm. Through deliberate attention to the breath and the practice of slow, deep breathing, people may trigger the body's relaxation response, which calms the nervous system and lessens sensations of tension and anxiety.

To engage in deep breathing exercises:

1. Take a seat comfortably in a chair with your hands resting on your lap or thighs and your feet flat on the ground.
2. Allow your attention to go inside by closing your eyes or lowering your gaze.
3. Take a long breath through your nose, filling your lungs with air and letting your abdomen stretch to its fullest.
4. Completely and slowly exhale through your lips, letting your abdomen softly contract as you do so.
5. Keep taking deep breaths and letting them out gently, paying attention to how the breath feels entering and leaving your body.

Assisted Visualization Tasks:

Using visualization to create a feeling of peace and well-being is known as guided imagery, and it is a technique for relaxing. People can induce a mental getaway from tension and anxiety by visualizing calm and serene situations or experiences, which encourages relaxation and stress reduction.

To put guided imagery into practice:

1. Locate a peaceful, cozy area where you may unwind without interruptions.
2. To calm your body and find your center, close your eyes and take a few deep breaths.
3. Envision a serene and quiet landscape in your thoughts, such as a calm beach, a verdant forest, or a serene garden.
4. As you lose yourself in the visualization, use all of your senses to take in the sights, sounds, scents, and feelings of the situation you've envisioned.
5. Give yourself permission to completely feel the calm and relaxation that results from the guided imagery practice, remaining in the present and releasing any stress or tension.

Chair Yoga Pose for Relaxation and Stress Reduction:

With the assistance of a chair, chair yoga provides a pleasant and accessible approach to performing stretches and yoga postures while seated. By releasing tight muscles, increasing circulation, and soothing the mind, these positions can aid in promoting relaxation, lowering stress levels, and relieving tension.

For relaxation and stress reduction, try these chair yoga poses:

1. Seated Forward Fold: Place your feet flat on the floor and sit up straight on a chair. Breathe in as your spine lengthens, and out as your hips pivot forward and your body folds over your thighs. Let your arms drop to the floor, or take hold of each other's elbows. Take a few deep breaths to hold, and then gently raise yourself back up.

2. Seated Cat-Cow Stretch: Place your hands on your knees while sitting tall on a chair. In the Cow Pose, inhale as you lift your chest toward the ceiling with your back arched; in the Cat Pose, exhale as you curve your spine and tuck your chin into your chest. Maintain a fluid transition between these two actions, matching each movement to your breathing.

3. Seated Spinal Twist: Place your feet flat on the ground while sitting tall on a chair. Breathe in as you extend your back and out as you turn your body to the right, with your right hand resting on the chair's back and your left hand resting on the outside of your right thigh. After holding for a few breaths, switch to the opposite side.

Including Relaxation Methods in Everyday Life:

To include chair yoga, guided visualization, and deep breathing exercises in your everyday routine:

- Schedule a certain period each day for relaxation techniques, such as right before bed, during a lunch break, or first thing in the morning.

- When faced with difficult circumstances or changes, as before a large presentation, during a hectic workday, or following a distressing encounter, use relaxation techniques to help manage stress.
Try out a variety of relaxation methods to see which one suits you the most. Don't be scared to combine or mix approaches for optimum impact.
- Remember that the advantages of practicing relaxation methods consistently over time tend to compound, so practice with patience.

To sum up, implementing relaxation methods into everyday living, such as chair yoga, guided imagery, and deep breathing, might be a useful strategy to lower stress, encourage relaxation, and improve general well-being. You may develop stronger stress resistance, enhance your capacity to handle obstacles, and have a greater feeling of balance and tranquility in your life by incorporating these techniques into your daily routine.

Exercises for Mental Fitness

Increasing Mental Health: Mind-Sharpening Activities

It's crucial to include mental fitness activities in your daily routine if you want to preserve cognitive function, enhance memory, and support general brain health. A few things that might help you maintain mental acuity include memory exercises, brain teasers, and mindfulness exercises. We'll talk about the advantages of these mental fitness activities in this session as well as the significance of giving mental health priority for general health.

Puzzles and Brain Games:

Playing brain games and solving puzzles is a great method to test your cognitive talents, activate your brain's neural connections, and maintain mental acuity. Playing games like Sudoku, logic puzzles, crosswords, and brain-training applications might assist in strengthening mental agility, memory retention, and problem-solving abilities.

By consistently putting riddles and brainteasers to the test, you can:

- Sharpen cognitive skills: Playing brain games makes you think critically, evaluate information, and make judgments fast. This improves mental clarity.
- Boost memory: Playing games and doing exercises centered around memory will help build brain connections that are linked to memory recall, which will improve knowledge retention and recall.
- Improve focus and concentration: Solving a puzzle or staying focused on a task needs prolonged attention and concentration, which can help you focus on daily chores more effectively.

Exercises for Memory:

Memory retention and recall-related cognitive processes are the focus of memory exercises. These exercises might be as basic as association and repetition or as sophisticated as memory games and mnemonic devices.

Here are a few instances of memory exercises:

- Visualization techniques: To assist knowledge being more efficiently encoded into memory, try seeing it in your mind's eye.
- Association exercises: To aid in memory retrieval, and establish relationships or linkages between new and prior knowledge.
- Recall exercises: Without consulting other sources, test your memory by asking you to recall names, lists, or other information.

Including memory exercises in your daily routine allows you to:

- Boost memory retention: Consistently engaging in memory-related activities can fortify the brain circuits linked to memory, ultimately resulting in enhanced knowledge retention over time.
- Improve cognitive function: Memory exercises make your brain work harder, which improves general brain health and cognitive function.
- Encourage brain plasticity: Memory exercises encourage neuroplasticity, which is the brain's capacity to modify and rearrange neural connections in reaction to novel stimuli and experiences.

The Significance of Mental Fitness in General Health and Welfare:

Because the mind and body are closely related, maintaining mental fitness is essential to overall health and well-being. Exercises for mental fitness enhance emotional and psychological health in addition to cognitive performance.

For general health, mental fitness is crucial for the following reasons:

- Cognitive health: Engaging in regular mental fitness activities might help lower the risk of neurodegenerative disorders like dementia and Alzheimer's as well as age-related cognitive decline.
- Emotional resilience: Mentally stimulating activities can help develop emotional resilience, strengthen coping mechanisms, and improve general mental health.
- Quality of life: As you age, retaining your independence, autonomy, and mental health is crucial to maintaining your quality of life.
- Lifelong learning: Engaging in mental fitness activities fosters intellectual curiosity and a lifetime of learning, which supports personal development and self-improvement.

In conclusion, preserving cognitive function, enhancing memory, and fostering general brain health require integrating mental fitness activities like brain games, puzzles, and memory exercises into your daily routine. You may live a longer and better life by keeping your mind active, maintaining intellectual curiosity, and placing a high priority on your mental health.

Chapter 8

Overcoming Typical Obstacles: Techniques for Maintaining Exercise Motivation

It can be difficult to stay motivated to work out on a regular basis when faced with hectic schedules, conflicting priorities, and boredom or exhaustion. However, people may overcome typical barriers and maintain their motivation to include exercise into their daily routine by putting effective tactics into practice and creating realistic objectives. We'll talk about how to maintain motivation in this session, including how to create both short- and long-term objectives and find delight in chair exercises.

Techniques for Motivation:

1. Determine Your Why: Knowing the reasons behind your desire to work out can help you stay motivated and goal-focused. Whether your goals are to achieve a certain fitness milestone, increase energy, lower stress, or improve your health, figuring out why you exercise can help you stay motivated to keep going.

2. Locate Your Inspirational Source: Look for motivational sources that speak to you. This might be

anything from reading about success stories to following fitness influencers on social media to being involved in a community of like-minded people. Being in the company of supportive people might help you stay motivated and responsible for achieving your objectives.

3. Establish a Supportive Environment: Put yourself in a setting that promotes and makes exercise easier. This may include setting up a specific area at home for exercise, finding a workout partner or enrolling in a fitness class, or planning workouts for when you're most likely to follow through.

4. Track Your Progress: Keeping track of your advancements and acknowledging your successes along the road will give you a sense of satisfaction and inspire you to keep moving forward. As you work toward your objectives, measure your progress and remain motivated by keeping a workout log, using fitness tracking apps, or setting milestones.

Creating both short- and long-term objectives:

1. Create SMART objectives: To guarantee responsibility and clarity, create objectives based on the SMART criteria: Specific, Measurable, Achievable, Relevant, and Time-bound. Deconstruct more ambitious objectives into more achievable smaller tasks or benchmarks, and set deadlines for each.

2. Prioritize Process objectives: Process objectives, which center on the activities and behaviors necessary to get those results, are more important than outcome-based goals (such as achieving a particular fitness level or reducing a certain amount of weight). For instance, setting a goal to work out a specific number of days a week or escalating the length or intensity of your sessions progressively over time.

3. Establish both immediate and long-term objectives: Long-term objectives that help you stay focused on the wider picture should be balanced with short-term objectives that offer instant satisfaction and feedback. While long-term objectives offer direction and purpose over time, short-term goals can support motivation and momentum in the short term.

Having Fun with Chair Exercises:

1. Explore Variety: By include a range of exercises and activities, you may make your chair workout regimen captivating and captivating. To keep things interesting and novel, try a variety of chair workouts, including sitting cardio, balance work, flexibility exercises, and strength training.

2. Play Music: To get you moving and improve your attitude while performing chair exercises, compile your favorite songs into a playlist that will motivate you to work out. Music has the power to uplift mood, divert

attention from discomfort, and increase drive to keep exercising.

3. Find Joy in Movement: Rather than thinking of exercise as a chore or a duty, concentrate on the feelings of movement and the advantages it offers to your body and mind. Seize the chance to use chair exercises to enhance your general well-being, decrease stress, and establish a stronger connection with your body.

4. Adjust and Modify: Don't be scared to change up your routine or workouts to fit your tastes and skill level. To ensure that your workouts are safe and pleasurable, pay attention to your body, respect your limitations, and make any modifications.

In conclusion, a mix of goal-setting methods, tactics, and discovering delight in your chosen activities are necessary to maintain your motivation to exercise on a regular basis. You may overcome typical obstacles and sustain long-term desire to prioritize your health and fitness by recognizing your reasons, developing SMART objectives, and investigating ways to make chair workouts pleasurable and rewarding.

Pain Control

Pain Management That Works: Reducing Soreness with Mild Motions

Managing pain, particularly joint pain, can be difficult and interfere with day-to-day activities. On the other hand, adding easy stretches and exercises to your regimen can help with pain and increase your range of motion. Prioritizing correct form and technique is essential to preventing more injuries, and for long-term health, it's critical to understand when to consult a doctor about chronic pain or discomfort. We'll talk about appropriate form and technique, efficient pain management techniques, and when to contact a doctor if pain or discomfort doesn't go away.

Modest Movements and Stretches to Reduce Joint Pain:

1. Range of Motion Exercises: Moderate range of motion exercises assist increase joint flexibility and reduce stiffness. Shoulder circles, wrist rolls, ankle circles, and neck rotations are a few examples. Execute these motions with grace and slowness, extending your range of motion to a comfortable point without pushing or straining.

2. Low-Impact Exercises: Without placing undue strain on the joints, low-impact exercises like swimming, cycling, and walking can assist increase joint mobility and lessen discomfort. To benefit from these activities, try to get in at least 30 minutes of moderate-intensity aerobic activity most days of the week.

3. Yoga and Tai Chi: These soft, low-impact exercise styles emphasize attentive breathing, flowing motions, and profound awareness. These exercises can lessen tension and encourage relaxation while also enhancing strength, flexibility, and balance. If you have mobility issues, try chair yoga or seated Tai Chi courses.

4. Stretching: To increase flexibility and lessen muscular tension, use mild stretching exercises in your regimen. Pay attention to your main muscle groups, including your calves, shoulders, back, hamstrings, and quads. For 15 to 30 seconds, hold each stretch while taking slow breaths and relaxing into the pose without jumping or using too much force.

The Significance of Correct Form and Method:

1. Preventing Injury: To avoid aggravating pre-existing pain and causing new injuries, proper form and technique are crucial. Be mindful of your alignment, posture, and muscle engagement when doing stretches or exercises to make sure you're not overstressing your joints or surrounding tissues.

2. Gradual Progression: As your strength and flexibility improves, start out slowly and progressively increase the time or intensity of your workouts. To prevent overexertion or damage, pay attention to your body's cues and refrain from pushing through pain or discomfort.

3. Seek Professional Advice: If you're not sure how to do a certain exercise, think about seeing a licensed physical therapist, fitness teacher, or other healthcare professional who can offer you individualized advice and assistance. They can assist you in creating an exercise regimen that is safe and suitable for your particular requirements and objectives.

When to Consult a Physician:

1. Persistent Pain or Discomfort: You should consult a doctor if your pain or discomfort is ongoing and doesn't go better with rest, light exercise, or over-the-counter pain relievers. This can indicate an injury or underlying medical problem that needs to be evaluated and treated by a specialist.

2. Sudden Increase in Pain: Stop exercising right once and get medical attention if you feel a sharp, stabbing pain during your exercise routine. This can be a sign of a fresh injury or an aggravation of an already-existing problem that requires immediate attention.

3. Limited Range of Motion: It's critical to consult a doctor to identify the cause and the best course of action if you observe a noticeable reduction in a joint's range of motion or mobility. A joint's limited range of motion may be the result of an injury, inflammation, or degenerative changes.

In summary, adding mild stretches and exercises to your daily regimen will help reduce joint discomfort and increase range of motion. Making good form and technique a priority is crucial to avoiding injuries and getting the most out of your workouts. It's essential to seek medical attention if you have ongoing pain or discomfort in order to determine the underlying reason and create a suitable treatment strategy. You may enhance your general quality of life and continue to lead an active lifestyle for years to come by being proactive about managing pain and giving joint health first priority.

Insufficient Time

Organizing Your Time Well: Fitting Chair Exercises Into Your Busy Schedule

It can be difficult to find time for exercise in today's hectic environment, especially when balancing obligations to your family, job, and other responsibilities. Even in times of limited time, you may maintain your health and level of activity by adding quick and efficient chair workouts to your regular routine. You may get beyond the obstacle of time constraints and enjoy the advantages of consistent physical activity by sprinkling exercise sessions throughout the day and making self-care a priority. In this talk, we'll look at how to fit chair workouts into a hectic schedule, how to conveniently divide up your workouts, and how important it is to prioritize taking care of yourself.

Including Quick and Powerful Chair Exercises:

1. Plan Ahead: Just as with any other meeting or obligation, fit quick workout breaks into your daily schedule. Select the times that are most convenient for you, whether it in the morning, right before bed, or during lunch breaks.

2. Put Efficiency First: Select chair workouts that are brief yet efficient, working several muscle groups and giving your entire body a workout in the shortest period of time. Seek for workouts that are easy to include into your everyday routine and require little room or equipment to do.

3. Maximize Intensity: Choose circuit-style training or high-intensity interval training (HIIT), which blend strength, cardio, and flexibility exercises into brief, intense bursts. These workouts are perfect for hectic schedules since they may yield the greatest results in the shortest amount of time.

4. Be Consistent: Even if you only exercise for a few minutes at a time, consistency is essential when it comes to adding exercise to your routine. To keep up the momentum and eventually see results, try to work out on a regular basis, even if it's only for ten to fifteen minutes at a time.

Dividing Workout Sessions During the Day:

1. Take Active Breaks: Throughout the day, take brief active breaks to stretch, exercise, and revitalize your body and mind as an alternative to spending extended amounts of time sitting. In order to break up with sedentary behavior, set reminders to get up, stretch, and take a short stroll every hour.

2. Employ Micro Workouts: Divide more extensive workouts into smaller, more doable chunks that you can accomplish all day. For instance, to get in 15 minutes of exercise, perform chair exercises for 5 minutes in the morning, 5 minutes at lunch, and 5 minutes at night.

3. Include Movement in Everyday chores: Seek ways to include movement in your regular activities and chores. For instance, park further away from your destination to gain extra steps, use the stairs rather than the elevator, or perform leg lifts or calf raises while on the phone or in line.

The Value of Making Self-Care a Priority:

1. Health Benefits: Regular exercise offers a host of advantages for both physical and mental health, such as better cardiovascular health, higher energy levels, a decrease in stress and anxiety, and an improvement in mood and general wellbeing. Making time for exercise

and putting self-care first may improve your physical and mental well-being as well as your general quality of life.

2. Stress Management: Exercise is an effective way to control stress and lessen the bad impacts of leading a busy life. Endorphins are neurotransmitters released during physical exercise that assist reduce stress and increase resilience by promoting sensations of enjoyment and relaxation.

3. Increased Productivity: By giving your brain a rest from constant cerebral duties and giving you a boost of energy and mental clarity, taking short pauses throughout the day to exercise can actually increase productivity and attention. You may maintain your alertness, attention, and productivity throughout the day by scheduling brief yet powerful chair exercise sessions into your calendar.

To sum up, time constraints often prevent people from exercising, but they don't have to prevent you from being healthy and happy. You may overcome the obstacle of time constraints and enjoy the advantages of consistent physical activity by adding quick and efficient chair workouts to your daily routine, spacing out your workouts throughout the day, and placing self-care first. Keep in mind that little things add up, so over time, even brief spurts of movement can result in noticeable gains in your fitness and general health.

Chapter 9:

Staying Active Outside of Chair Exercises

Including Movement in Everyday Life: Strategies for Continuing to Be Active During the Day

To preserve general health and well-being in today's sedentary environment, finding methods to include exercise in everyday life is crucial. A regular exercise routine, whether it be easy or involves focused movement, may make a big difference in one's physical, mental, and emotional well-being. We'll talk about how to keep moving throughout the day, why it's important to move often for general health, and easy exercises you can do whether sitting, standing, or walking.

Advice for Maintaining Your Daily Activity Level:

1. use Reminders: To help you remember to take breaks and exercise throughout the day, use alarms or calendar reminders. Set a reminder to break up extended periods of sitting every hour by standing up, stretching, or going for a little stroll.

2. Take activity intervals: Move and stretch your body during brief activity intervals rather than prolonged periods of sitting. To increase blood flow and mental

rejuvenation, take a few minutes to perform chair exercises, stroll about your house or workplace, or stand up and stretch.

3. Include Movement in Everyday Tasks: Seek ways to include movement in your everyday routine. If you can, walk or bike to work, utilize the stairs rather than the elevator, or move your body by doing housework like gardening or sweeping.

4. Make Exercise Fun: Choose some enjoyable things to incorporate into your daily schedule. Making movement enjoyable may help you stay motivated and involved, whether you're dancing to your favorite music, playing with your children or pets, or attending a group fitness class with friends.

Frequent Movement Is Essential for General Health:

1. Better Physical Health: Being physically active regularly helps you stay in a healthy weight range, lowers your chance of developing chronic conditions like diabetes, cancer, and heart disease, and generally increases your strength, flexibility, and physical fitness.

2. Improved Mental Health: Research has demonstrated that engaging in physical exercise may yield several advantages for mental health, such as lowering stress, anxiety, and depressive symptoms, elevating mood and

self-worth, and augmenting mental acuity and cognitive performance.

3. Enhanced Energy Levels: Engaging in regular physical activity enhances energy levels by augmenting blood circulation and oxygen transportation to the brain and muscles, diminishing exhaustion and sluggishness, and fostering a sensation of liveliness and wellness.

4. Better Sleep: By assisting in the regulation of sleep-wake cycles, lowering stress and anxiety levels, and encouraging relaxation and restfulness, regular physical exercise can enhance both the length and quality of sleep.

Easy Exercises You Can Perform While Walking, Standing, or Sitting:

1. When seated:
    - Seated Leg Raises: Raise one leg off the ground, erect it in front of you, and then return it to the starting position. On the opposite leg, repeat.
    - Marching while seated: Raise your knees to your chest and move your legs in a marching manner.
    - Seated Shoulder Rolls: To reduce stress and increase range of motion, roll your shoulders forward and backward in a circular manner.

2. When standing: - Calf Raises: Place your feet hip-width apart, lift yourself onto your toes, and then drop yourself back down.

Squats: Place your feet hip-width apart, bend your knees, and lower your hips back to the floor like you're sitting in a chair. Then, stand back up.
- Side Leg Lifts: Maintaining a straight leg, raise one leg to the side and then bring it back down while standing tall. Continue on the opposite side.

3. When you're walking, try these tips: - Brisk Walking: Walk faster to raise your heart rate and burn more calories.
- Interval Walking: To add variation and intensity to your stroll, alternate between intervals of fast walking and slower, recovery walking.
- Include steps: Look for opportunities to ascend steps while out on a stroll to mix things up a little and work various muscle groups.

In summary, sustaining general health and well-being requires incorporating activity into daily life. You may improve your physical and mental health as well as your quality of life by implementing these basic workouts into your daily routine, emphasizing frequent movement, and remaining active throughout the day. Always keep in mind that movement counts, so take advantage of the chance to exercise your body in ways that you find pleasurable and sustainable.

Taking Up Outdoor Activities: Using Nature to Improve Health and Well-Being

There are several advantages to participating in outdoor activities for one's physical, mental, and emotional health. Engaging in outdoor activities such as gardening, Tai Chi, or Qigong in a park, or taking a stroll in the fresh air and sunshine all offer chances to bond with the natural world, de-stress, and enhance general well-being. We'll talk about the advantages of outdoor activities and how they may all lead to a happier and healthier life in this conversation.

Strolling outside in the sunshine and fresh air:

One of the easiest yet most beneficial types of exercise is walking outside. It offers a host of health advantages as well as a chance to take in the scenery and rekindle one's connection with the natural world. The following are a few advantages of walking outside:

1. Physical Well-Being: Walking outside is a low-impact workout that promotes cardiovascular health, bone and muscular strength, and weight maintenance. Walking regularly can also lower your chance of developing chronic illnesses including diabetes, heart disease, and stroke.

2. Mental Health: Being outside in the sunshine and with clean air can be beneficial for mental health. It has been demonstrated that taking a walk outdoors may enhance mood and self-esteem, lower stress, anxiety, and sadness, and improve mental health in general.

3. Connection with Nature: Going for a stroll outside gives you the chance to see and feel the beauty of nature. Being in nature, whether it be by taking a stroll in a park, along a beach, or through a forest, may help lower stress levels and foster a sense of calm and serenity.

Using Gardens as a Type of Exercise:

Not only is gardening a fulfilling pastime, but it's also a type of exercise with several health advantages. Whether you grow herbs, veggies, or flowers, gardening gives you a chance to get outside, move, and establish a connection with the land. The following are a few advantages of gardening:

1. **Activities Physically:** Digging, planting, weeding, and watering are just a few of the physical tasks involved with gardening that enhance strength, flexibility, and endurance. Gardening is a great way to increase general fitness and burn calories.

2. Stress Reduction: By fostering a sense of achievement, fostering a connection with nature, and encouraging present-moment awareness, gardening has been demonstrated to lower stress and encourage relaxation.

Taking care of plants and seeing them flourish can be a gratifying and healing experience.

3. Mental Well-Being: By encouraging mindfulness, lowering anxiety and depressive symptoms, and enhancing general mood and well-being, gardening can improve mental health. Taking care of plants and being in an environment full of greenery may make one feel happy and at ease.

Qigong or Tai Chi in a Park or Other Outdoor Setting:

Ancient Chinese mind-body exercises called Qigong and Tai Chi include deep breathing, meditation, and soft, flowing motions. Tai Chi and Qigong may be practiced outside in a park or other natural location, which can increase their advantages and foster a closer relationship with the natural world. The following are some advantages of Qigong and Tai Chi:

1. Physical Health: Qigong and Tai Chi improve posture and coordination, balance, strength, and flexibility. They also improve cardiovascular health. Especially for elderly persons, deliberate, unhurried motions can help lower the risk of falls and injury.

2. Stress Reduction: Tai Chi and Qigong are great ways to relieve stress since they ease mental strain, ease physical tension, and encourage relaxation. Stress and

anxiety may be reduced and the mind can become quieter by concentrating on breathing and movement.

3. Mind-Body Connection: Qigong and Tai Chi encourage a strong mental-physical bond that leads to inner serenity, harmony, and balance. This connection may be strengthened by practicing outside in a natural environment, giving practitioners a stronger sense of rootedness and earthiness.

In conclusion, engaging in outdoor pursuits like walking, gardening, and park Tai Chi or Qigong offers a host of advantages for mental, emotional, and physical health. Taking in the sunshine and clean air, spending time in nature, or practicing moderate exercise and meditation are all opportunities to nurture the body, mind, and spirit. Including outdoor activities in your daily routine may make your life happier, healthier, and more satisfying.

Social Interaction

Promoting Social Interaction: Improving Physical Activity with Relationships

Working out doesn't have to be done alone. Engaging in physical activity alongside friends and family, joining a local senior exercise class or group, and taking part in virtual exercise classes and online communities are all great methods to prioritize physical health and promote social interaction. We'll go over the advantages of each strategy and how they affect responsibility, motivation, and general well-being in this conversation.

Enrolling in a Local Senior Exercise Program or Club:

1. Community Connection: Enrolling in a senior fitness class or organization in your area gives you the chance to meet people who have similar interests and aspirations. These seminars frequently promote a feeling of support and camaraderie, fostering an environment where participants may uplift and inspire one another.

2. organized Exercise: Most senior fitness programs include organized workouts taught by certified instructors who can modify the routines to suit each student's requirements and skill level. This guarantees that participants experience the social advantages of group exercise in addition to receiving safe and helpful exercise coaching.

3. Accountability: Consistency and accountability in your workout regimen may be improved by regularly attending courses. Exercise becomes more important and you are more likely to adhere to your fitness objectives when you know that people are counting on you to show up.

Working Out With Friends or Family:

1. Inspiration and Support: Working out with loved ones may offer inspiration and encouragement, which can help you stick to your fitness objectives. Exercise routine adherence, accountability, and enjoyment can all be enhanced by working out with a partner.

2. Quality Time: In addition to enhancing physical health, exercising with loved ones provides an opportunity for quality time spent together. Working out with friends or family may improve relationships and make enduring memories, whether you go for a stroll, a bike ride, or take a fitness class together.

3. Variety and Fun: Working out with others gives you the chance to try out new things and mix up your routines. Fitness may be made more fun and interesting by working out with friends or family, whether it's through a new activity, game, or outdoor experience.

Digital Fitness Courses and Online Forums:

1. Accessibility: From the comforts of home, virtual fitness courses and online groups offer easy access to fitness materials and support. People may engage in fitness programs more easily because of this accessibility, regardless of their schedule or location.

2. Variety of Options: A vast array of fitness courses and programs are available on virtual platforms to accommodate a range of interests, tastes, and fitness levels. In the realm of online fitness, there is something

for everyone, regardless of your interests in yoga, dancing, strength training, or aerobic exercises.

3. Connection and Accountability: Engaging in online groups and virtual fitness classes enables people to meet like-minded people, exchange experiences, and offer assistance and motivation to one another. This sensation of belonging to a group can improve commitment to a fitness regimen, motivation, and accountability.

To sum up, social interaction is essential for improving workout experiences and advancing general well-being. Greater motivation, accountability, and pleasure of exercise can result from interacting with people while placing a priority on physical health. This can be achieved via joining a local senior exercise class or group, working out with friends or family, or taking part in virtual exercise classes and online communities. People may attain their fitness objectives and enhance their overall quality of life by creating meaningful relationships and social support networks.

Chapter 10

When to Think About Senior Chair Exercises

Maintaining one's physical health and mobility as one age is crucial to one's overall wellbeing. Traditional exercise regimens might be difficult for many seniors because of conditions including joint discomfort, balance problems, or decreased mobility. In these situations, chair exercises provide a secure and useful substitute to support elders in maintaining their independence and level of activity. It's important to know the advantages of chair exercises for seniors as well as the telltale indicators of whether they're appropriate.

Advantages of Chair Exercises for Elderly People

1. Minimal Effect:
Chair exercises are great for seniors with arthritis or other musculoskeletal issues since they are easy on the joints and lower the chance of harm.
2. Enhanced Circulation
Seated exercises improve blood flow and lower the risk of circulation-related problems including varicose veins and blood clots.
3. Increased Dexterity and Strength:
Seniors who regularly engage in chair exercises can enhance their flexibility and muscular strength, both of

which are critical for preserving mobility and averting falls.

4. Improved Balance and Posture:
In order to assist elders in maintaining good posture and lowering their risk of falling, many chair exercises emphasize core strength and balance.

5. Mental Health:
Seniors who engage in physical exercise are less likely to experience depression and cognitive impairment since it has been related to better mood and cognitive performance.

Signs Seniors Should Think About Chair Exercises:

1. Restricted Movement:
Chair exercises help seniors who have trouble standing or walking for long periods to be seated and yet get physical activity.

2. Joint Pain:
Traditional workouts might be difficult or uncomfortable if you have arthritis or other joint-related conditions. Chair workouts provide a means of maintaining an active lifestyle without aggravating joint pain.

3. Problems with Equilibrium:
Chair exercises that target stability and coordination might be beneficial for seniors who struggle with balance or who fear falling.

4. Rehabilitating:

Seniors may need to progressively restore strength and mobility after surgery or an injury. Chair exercises can offer a regulated and secure rehabilitative setting.

5. A Sedentary Way of Life

Sedentary lifestyles can cause muscular weakness and decreased flexibility in seniors. They might become more used to physical activity by learning chair exercises.

In summary:

Seniors may maintain their physical and mental well-being and keep active with chair exercises, which are adaptable and easily accessible. Caregivers, medical professionals, and seniors themselves may make well-informed decisions about introducing chair exercises into their daily routine by being aware of the advantages of these exercises and the telltale signals that suggest when they are appropriate. Chair exercises can help seniors of all fitness levels age well and live better lives by either serving as their main source of exercise or as an addition to other activities.

Evaluating Physical Restrictions
Evaluating Physical Restrictions: Recognizing Mobility Problems and Standing Exercise Dangers

Seniors must continue to remain physically active to maintain their general well-being, independence, and mobility. To guarantee that exercise is both safe and beneficial, it's equally critical to recognize and evaluate physical limitations. This entails figuring out which mobility problems call for sitting workouts and which situations might make standing activities risky.

Recognizing Mobility Problems:

1. restricted range of motion
Seniors who struggle with activities requiring standing or dynamic motions may be limited in their range of motion in their joints. They can work within their comfortable range without putting undue strain on their joints by doing workouts while seated.
2. Issues with Equilibrium:
Seniors with poor balance are more likely to fall when performing standing activities. Exercises performed while seated offer a secure basis, lowering the chance of falls and enabling seniors to concentrate on building strength and flexibility without worrying about being hurt.
3. Joint Pain:
Pain and discomfort during weight-bearing activities can be caused by joint-related disorders such as osteoporosis and arthritis. Because they put less strain on the joints, seated activities are more suited for elderly people with persistent discomfort.
4. Fatigue or Weakness:
Standing exercises might be difficult for seniors who are weak or tired from age, disease, or medication. A milder option that enables individuals to safely and gradually increase their strength is to engage in seated activities.
5. After Surgery or Trauma:

Seniors may experience temporary or permanent movement limits after surgery or an injury, necessitating adjustments to their exercise regimen. Seniors who participate in seated exercises can continue their physical activity during their recovery and benefit from a regulated rehabilitation setting.

Recognizing the Dangers of Standing Exercises:

1. Fall Hazard:
When performing standing activities, seniors who struggle with balance or mobility are more likely to fall and sustain severe injuries including fractures or brain damage.

2. Overdoing it:
Particularly for seniors with less endurance or stamina, standing activities may demand more energy and effort than seated exercises. Fatigue, strained muscles, and other problems may result from overexertion.

3. Joint Stress:
Seniors with arthritis or other joint-related disorders may experience more pain and suffering from weight-bearing activities because they place more strain on their joints.

4. Feeling lightheaded or dizzy:
When rising fast, seniors may feel lightheaded or dizzy, especially if they take drugs that influence their blood circulation or have low blood pressure. Seniors who engage in seated activities are kept in a steady position, which reduces the chance of these symptoms.

5. Safety Issues:

Seniors may find it more difficult to maintain balance and coordination when performing activities while standing, which raises the possibility of falling or losing control of their motions. Exercises done while seated provide a safer option with a lower chance of harm.

In summary:

Seniors can be effectively and safely engaged in physical activity by evaluating their physical limitations and being aware of the hazards involved with standing activities. Exercise programs may be customized to match the requirements and capacities of elders by caregivers, healthcare experts, and seniors themselves by detecting mobility limitations that may need sitting exercises and recognizing when standing activities offer a risk of injury. For seniors of all fitness levels, exercise should always be done carefully and changed as necessary, whether one is sitting or standing. This will ensure everyone's safety and optimize the advantages.

seeking medical advice before beginning a new fitness program.
Taking Care of Medical Conditions

Taking Care of Health Issues Before Beginning a New Workout Program

People must speak with a healthcare professional before starting a new fitness program, particularly if they have any underlying medical concerns. Before beginning an exercise program, it is important to address any health issues. This includes evaluating any chronic diseases, previous operations, or injuries, and customizing activities to meet individual needs.

Chronic Illnesses:

1. arthritic
People who have arthritis frequently have stiffness and soreness in their joints, which makes doing high-impact workouts difficult. Because chair exercises offer a low-impact means of enhancing joint mobility and muscle strength without aggravating pain, they can be very helpful.
2. The disease osteoporosis
Osteoporosis in seniors causes brittle bones that are more prone to breaking. Exercises involving weight bearing, like walking or standing, may make injuries more likely. By lessening the strain on bones, chair workouts provide a safer substitute while still increasing muscular strength and bone density.

Rehabilitation After an Injury or Surgery:

1. Following Surgery:
People may need to progressively resume physical exercise after surgery to promote healing. Because chair exercises allow for regulated motions and minimum

impact on healing tissues, they might be a great alternative throughout the rehabilitation process.

2. Rehabilitating After Injury:

Customized exercises can assist people in regaining strength and flexibility while lowering their risk of reinjury, whether they are recuperating from a sprain, strain, or other injury. Chair exercises are safe and effective ways to target particular muscle groups and range of motion during rehabilitation.

Customizing Exercises for Particular Health Needs:

1. Tailored Programs:

Healthcare professionals can collaborate with patients to create customized exercise regimens that meet their unique fitness objectives and health concerns. This might entail choosing suitable chair exercises, adapting motions to account for restrictions, and escalating intensity gradually as tolerated.

2. Tracking Development:

To guarantee ongoing improvement and avoid injuries, training regimens must be regularly reviewed and adjusted. Healthcare professionals may evaluate each person's response to exercise and adjust as necessary to maximize results.

3. Teaching about Security:

To teach people about safe exercise practices, such as appropriate form, and pace, and identifying the early warning indicators of overexertion or injury, providers are essential. Providers may assist persons in engaging in physical exercise safely and confidently by arming them with information and direction.

In summary:

People must speak with a healthcare professional before starting a new fitness program to treat any underlying medical issues and customize activities to fit their particular needs. Chair exercises are a flexible and accessible solution for people of all abilities, whether they are treating chronic ailments like osteoporosis or arthritis, recuperating from surgery or an injury, or just looking to enhance general fitness. People can start a safe and efficient fitness program that improves the quality of life and physical health with the right direction and oversight from healthcare professionals.

Recognizing Age-Related Shifts: Modifying Fitness Programs for Seniors

Many physiological changes that occur with age might affect an individual's strength, balance, and flexibility. Understanding these age-related changes is essential to creating fitness regimens that support general health and well-being and adapt to the changing demands of elders. It's crucial to accept chair workouts as a secure and reliable alternative for elders to deal with these alterations and guarantee ongoing physical activity.

Identifying Changes Related to Age:

1. Reduced Mass of Muscle:
As people age, their muscular mass gradually decreases, which results in a loss of strength and power. Elderly people may find it harder to do tasks that involve lifting or carrying things, and they may become tired more easily when they push themselves physically.

2. Deficiency in Balance:
Seniors who have eyesight, inner ear, or proprioceptive changes may have trouble maintaining their balance and stability. This raises the possibility of accidents and falls, especially while engaging in activities that call for walking or standing on uneven ground.

3. Diminished Adaptability
Two major age-related changes that might impact flexibility are reduced range of motion and tight joints. Elderly people may have trouble bending, reaching, or doing stretches, which can cause pain and limited movement.

4. Reduced Reaction Time:
Cognitive function, particularly coordination and response speed, can also be impacted by aging. Seniors are more likely to have accidents or falls because they may find it harder to react rapidly to changes in their surroundings.

5. Decrease in Bone Density:
Age-related bone loss and osteoporosis can weaken bones, increasing their vulnerability to fractures. To preserve bone density and lower their risk of fractures,

seniors may need to adjust their exercise regimens to incorporate weight-bearing exercises.

The Value of Modifying Exercise Programs:

1. Customized Method:
Seniors' unique requirements and limitations might be catered to in fitness regimens created with their age in mind. Exercises that focus on strength, balance, and flexibility can help seniors maintain or enhance their physical function and level of independence.

2. Minimizing Risk:
Exercise regimen modifications lower the chance of falls, injuries, and other unfavorable aging-related occurrences. Particularly chair exercises provide elders with a safe, supervised setting to exercise while reducing the chance of mishaps.

3. Enhanced Life Quality:
Seniors who engage in regular physical activity benefit greatly from enhanced mood, enhanced cognitive function, and enhanced general well-being. Seniors can continue to experience these advantages and keep their independence as they age by customizing their exercise regimens to suit their changing demands.

4. Extended Health:
Seniors who exercise to address age-related changes might lessen the effects of chronic illnesses including osteoporosis, arthritis, and cardiovascular disease. Regular exercise can lengthen life, lower the chance of problems, and assist control of symptoms.

5. Increased Capability of Function:

Seniors who follow modified exercise regimens can preserve or increase their functional ability, which makes it easier and more confident for them to carry out everyday tasks. This encourages independence, empowerment, and self-sufficiency.

Chair Exercises for Embracing:

1. Secure and Easily Reachable:
For seniors of all fitness levels and abilities, chair exercises provide a secure and convenient alternative. Chairs give seniors the support and stability they need to do a range of activities without worrying about falling or being hurt.
2. Flexible and Powerful:
Chair workouts are excellent for a wide range of people since they can be tailored to target different muscle areas and fitness objectives. Chairs offer a flexible platform for encouraging physical activity and functional health, ranging from mild stretches to workouts focused on increasing strength.
3. Comfortable and Convenient:
Chair exercises are a practical option for seniors who may not have easy access to fitness facilities or mobility. They may be performed in almost any place. Seated positions also ease joint and muscular tension, adding to the comfort and enjoyment of activities.
4. Participation in Society:

Chair exercises are a great way to foster camaraderie and social contact whether done alone or in a group. Support, encouragement, and a feeling of community are provided by group programs, which can improve motivation and consistency in following an exercise program.

In summary:

Creating fitness regimens that suit seniors' changing demands and advance their best health and well-being requires an understanding of age-related changes in strength, balance, and flexibility. Seniors may address these changes and reap the many advantages of regular physical activity by embracing chair exercises as a secure and practical solution. Older persons' quality of life can be improved and healthy aging can be supported by caregivers, healthcare providers, and seniors themselves by including chair exercises in fitness programs and modifying exercise regimens to account for age-related changes.

Made in the USA
Las Vegas, NV
17 May 2025

22309142R00075